I HAVE THE NEXT TEN MILLION YEARS TO LIE STILL-NOW IS THE TIME TO MOVE

A SIMPLE NO NONSENSE GUIDE HOW TO CHANGE YOUR LIFE FOR THE BETTER

ERIC SOLOMON

authorHOUSE®

AuthorHouse™ UK
1663 Liberty Drive
Bloomington, IN 47403 USA
www.authorhouse.co.uk
Phone: UK TFN: 0800 0148641 (Toll Free inside the UK)
UK Local: (02) 0369 56322 (+44 20 3695 6322 from outside the UK)

Published by AuthorHouse 05/17/2023

ISBN: 979-8-8230-8260-0 (sc)
ISBN: 979-8-8230-8261-7 (e)

Library of Congress Control Number: 2023908998

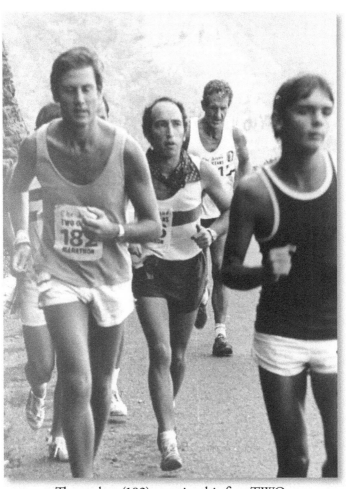

The author (182) running his first TWO OCEANS marathon-1975

DEDICATED TO THOSE WHO FEEL THEY
CAN'T DO IT - I'VE GOT NEWS FOR YOU-
YOU CAN !

CONTENTS

FOREWORD

It has been said that the sixties and seventies in South Africa were the golden years of medicine. I can concur. I was fortunate to have grown up in South Africa and privileged to be able to attend a top class medical school, an opportunity unfortunately generally not afforded to non caucasians at the time, which forever will remain a blight on South Africa's checkered past and unfortunately future I dare say.

But this book is not about politics, a subject I am not particularly fond of. I have always found myself to be critical of whoever is in power because I have never witnessed anywhere a government fulfilling its promises and obligations to the people who voted them in. Instead I will write about something where I was able to make a difference and bring about change in my life and the lives of those willing to take a chance in trying out my suggestions.

We are not born with knowledge, it has to be acquired from life's experiences. Sometimes the lessons of life are blatantly obvious but sometimes it takes effort to see the 'not so obvious'. We are inclined to believe what is comfortable for us and shun advice that might cause uneasiness, the path less travelled. Rarely do we unequivocally accept advice which we disagree with and as a result, we are left at the end of the day with uncertainty on many crucial matters in our lives. Good health for instance is quintessential in our lives, yet we are still uncertain of which path to follow in order to achieve this. Long standing universally accepted standards are being overturned causing uneasiness. Standards are no longer being accepted and are challenged continuously. One no longer knows what is true. The lines of discernment are blurred.

During my training as a medical doctor, we were taught to be vigilant and observant, which became second nature. I mention this specifically, as it is vital in understanding how our perceptions have changed particularly in the medical field which has allowed a culture of slovenliness to develop for lack of a more appropriate description.

Having spent a considerable portion of my life in the practice of medicine I learned many things that certainly influenced my life considerably. Had I not learned something from my profession, then, as stated in Ecclesiastes, all would have been in vain. Yet I often gave advice to patients but failed to apply the same advice to myself.

It must be remembered that I practiced as a general practitioner in South Africa in a relatively small town during the early seventies when we lacked the expertise and equipment of today. That's not to say that we were totally in the dark, but rather that we relied more on our senses and common sense.

Today's sceptics imply that old practices and ideas from the past are archaic and no longer have a place in modern medicine and are therefore irrelevant. It is said that modern science supersedes the old theories. It is here that I take umbrage because not everything coming out of research today can be trusted and certainly not all from the past should be relegated. The Covid pandemic a case in point. I will allude to this later.

Where am I going with this?

With this book I want to detail my experiences on a personal level which often involved several hotly contested subjects which I have tackled head-on, often finding myself in direct conflict and directly opposed to the popular trends of the day. Some are as obvious as the proverbial elephant in the room, others not so.

In part one I will discuss my own epiphany which was life changing, leading me on a path I so easily could have missed. In part two I will concentrate more on the nutritional side of my epiphany. I don't profess to be an expert in nutrition nor running by any means, but what I will do though is present to the reader regimes I discovered throughout the years, which I adopted and applied to my own eating habits some of which especially these days run contrary to the latest fads. I call my discovery a 'stroke of serendipity'.

For the sake of simplicity, I have divided the book into two parts. Part one describes my discovery of running, and part two is concerned with the diets I have developed and adopted over the years.

Eric Solomon,
Brunskog,
Sweden

May, 2023

PART ONE

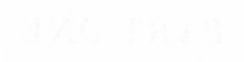

WHERE IT ALL STARTED

Having returned from working in London as a senior house officer at one of London's six teaching hospitals at the time, St. Mary's in Praed Street, I entered the world of general practice in Benoni, a town of 55,000 inhabitants in 1970. I had passed the final MBChB exam in 1968 at the university of Pretoria, then spent the next year as a houseman (intern) in Boksburg at an 850 bed hospital, where I was fortunate to acquire much 'hands on' experience, vital for going into GP in South Africa, where one would be expected to be able to handle uncomplicated general surgery and obstetrics with alacrity despite not being specialised in those two disciplines per se. The need for expertise far outstrips the supply and has continued down the slippery slope as the population swells unabated.

Initially GP proved to be ideal. The size of the town was adequate, being situated some 20 miles from the centre of the gold reef, namely Johannesburg where every whim could be satisfied not available in our town.

There were five partners in our practice, and each had his own forte, which when put together was a formidable group practice in deed. We were virtually able to handle most medical and surgical emergencies, not to mention the run of the mill general practice cases seen in any practice.

Despite there being six of us the workload was very heavy, a problem of our own making. We allowed patients to pitch up to our surgery without booking an appointment which often meant working extremely long hours. I joined the practice knowing this, but unfortunately didn't really understand the implications thereof. Working in a practice with sometimes serious responsibilities and decisions to be made was some undertaking which didn't take long to sink in. Nevertheless the work was enjoyable albeit stressful at times.

After a long night on duty without the previous or next day free to recover, was telling even from early days in the practice. Similarly working an entire weekend and then being ready to begin the next day supposedly fresh and able, was not conducive to a happy family life. With an ever demanding and increasing patient load the situation was not going to improve any time soon.

There was an ever decreasing amount of time for exercise, and before I knew it, my day consisted solely of working, coming home in the evenings, eating dinner and then falling into bed exhausted, only to be woken by the alarm clock to start the next day. I seemed to be always tired and exhausted and was totally oblivious of what food I was putting into my mouth. The weight gain was surreptitious and stealth-like, and I was completely oblivious to the changes taking place in my body, and too busy to recognise the steady decline in my relationship with my immediate family.

I continued giving patients the usual advice regarding weight loss, but never once applying the advice to myself.

I'd blab out the usual mantra of eat less and exercise more. I don't ever recall any success with this formula then and now. It took me a long time to realise that people are generally not interested in hard work and applying restraint to cure an ailment when there is pharmacology available to do the job pain free.

LESSON 1: *there is no pain free way to lose weight or get fit!*

The early seventies was not a period where masses of people were seen to be exercising in parks or gyms. The sort of activities seen on weekends would be a game of cricket on the village green, a tussle between two lowly places teams batting it out, with a few enthusiasts watching with beer in hand under the oak trees prevalent around most cricket pitches in those days, a perfectly civilised thing to do. International competitions were few and far between. TV was not yet introduced into South Africa, only arriving in 1976. The radio would have to suffice for a few more years till TV finally arrived.

Besides this lack of sport on TV, there was a dearth of equipment particularly in the field of running, so even if one wanted to pursue the not so gentle and not yet popular sport of running, the only shoes available at the time were tennis shoes, offering zero support for the potential marathoner. Tennis rackets were certainly available and there were a few courts scattered around town and I was lucky to have friends who possessed one. Thursday evenings was the chosen night and when not on duty, I was fortunate to get in a few sets, although as it turned out I wasn't very good but enjoyed the fellowship all the same.

Life as a small town doctor had its advantages. One could say we were a like a big fish in a small tank. In those days doctors were respected to a point but the way the fees were structured left a lot to be desired. There were serious disadvantages as well. Payment by the medical aids went back to the patient and then passed on to us if we were lucky. This was cumbersome and unsatisfactory, working hard and getting poorly remunerated by an imperfect system.

Overall I was satisfied but felt that I was getting into a groove. I was far from fit, something I always managed to be during my time at university albeit never very fit. Despite playing low league rugger at medical school, and then, as was the norm, imbibing vast amounts of beer after the game I never paid attention to my weight as it always seemed to be constant. It was not exactly the sort of thing medical students prioritised in those days However the inevitable happened and my weight started creeping up surreptitiously as it tends to do after the age of 25 years.

Dented ego

It transpired one day after finishing off at the surgery that I came home, to find my wife in conversation with our good looking neighbour. However any notion of an exchange of pleasantries was abruptly ended. Nothing is more damaging to a man's ego than being told by a beautiful woman that his belly is disgusting! Imagine the jolt! That memory was indelibly etched into my brain forever, life would never be the same again.

The heavy mood hung over me for a few days it must be said. Could anything be done about this I wondered? I had never considered dieting, it was only for patients. Besides diets rarely worked I told myself. I learned to live with the situation. All I needed to do was avoid the good looking neighbour and if we did meet, I'd need to pull my stomach in. By the way, abdominoplasties were not yet in vogue in our neck of the woods not that I would ever have considered the procedure.

EPIPHANY

Our general practice had two surgeries, the main one situated in the central part of town and the other was in the so-called industrial sites, situated close to all the factories, where we could manage the injuries and acute illnesses of the workers. The partners in the practice rotated through both surgeries on a daily basis and the system worked well.

During 1972 in South Africa there was a campaign to increase the wellbeing of the population by encouraging moderate exercise in the form of walking. Jingles were heard on the radio throughout the day and billboards were often seen on the side of the roads.

On one particular evening after leaving the industrial surgery for my last session of the day in town, I was feeling particularly lethargic and could easily have called it a day and headed off home, but that was out go the question.

On the way to the surgery my eye caught sight of a newly erected billboard which screamed out its message loud and clear-

"WALK FOR YOUR LIFE, AND WHEN YOU ARE NOT WALKING-DRIVE A DATSUN !"

This add made me sit up and think as never before, but I

was yet to receive the final insult later that day which would change my life forever. This would happen shortly.

On reaching the surgery, I went to the back room to leave my doctors bag to be replenished by one of our nurses as was the routine ready for use the next day.

I had five patients to examine, the last one being a young man needing a routine medical examination for insurance purposes as he was applying for a new job. The nurse who was to pack my medical bag, came in with the patient's physical measurements and urine analysis results. She laid them on my desk and left with the following exclamation-

"This bloke is overweight-shocking to see how they let themselves go!"

The examination didn't yield anything abnormal (or so I thought), so I sent him merrily on his way.

Finally the day was over and I could go home. I took one more look at the form I had just filled in to see if all the details were correct. I noticed that we both were exactly the same height, six foot three and three quarter inches or 193 centimetres tall. I then looked closely at his weight, it was 198 pounds (90 kg). I stepped on the scale nervously and slowly glanced down in trepidation fearing the worst. My fears were well founded as the scale showed 202 pounds (92 kg). Surely not!

This was the first time I had stood on a scale since leaving school where my weight was 176 pounds(80kg). Surely I could not have gained 26 pounds (almost12 kg) without noticing it? If it weren't for two rude awakenings who knows where I might have ended up? I closed my bag and headed for home.

I walked in to our apartment which was in a large

complex of apartments which filled an entire block. I informed my wife that I was going to go for a run with Claude, our neighbour on the other side, except he was unaware of my hair-brain idea. I needed support and it was to come from Claud.

As stated previously running gear was primitive and I was going to run in tennis shoes and a thick dark track suit, which would help keep my apparently ungainly body profile hidden. Fortunately it was dusk and the light was fast fading. Claude's wife and mine stood together shaking their heads in disbelief as we set off into the impending darkness wondering if we had lost our senses.

We set of at what felt like a fast pace but in reality was extremely slow, we were simply not capable of any speed. I managed to run a mere 300 meters, when every part of my body screamed out for me to stop. My lungs were at their limits, with that taste of blood in my mouth most beginners know too well. My knees were at breaking point or so it felt. There was no way I was going to run around the entire complex. I had set my sights far to high. Clearly not only was I not looking good, but I was far from being in any shape to speak of. A physical and mental refurbishment was called for and could wait no longer. Could it be done ?

Claude took strain at being bludgeoned into having to accompanying me and I realised it was selfish of me to drag him along, but I give him credit for continuing albeit for a few months till sanity once more prevailed. I mention Claude because we had a mutual friend Ronnie, a good few years older than me. I was 28 years old at the time and Ronnie was 39. We decided to invite Ronnie to join us on one of our runs to which he surprisingly agreed. We were stunned to see the 'old' man arrive and literally run us into the ground. I had no idea that Ronnie was this good or that we were so bad.

The three of us struck up a running relationship and so started a long and lasting friendship which would take Ronnie and myself on an unimaginable running journey lasting many years despite our future paths leading us to reside on opposite sides of the globe.

STRETCHING OUR GOALS

Initially we set out to try and run one mile without stopping. This took me longer than I imagined it would. I suffered with panful knees for about three weeks and then the discomfort fortunately subsided. At this early stage we were introduced to an amazing fellow, Manie Alberts, a physiotherapist in town who was blind from the age of 18 months, but otherwise in outstandingly good health and shape. Manie assured me that my knee pain was 'normal' for beginners and would sooner or later pass. In retrospect the knee pain was termed anterior knee pain or chondromalasia of the patella, which is extremely common in new runners. Apparently if I persisted through this injury according to Manie, without ingesting medication, I stood a chance of becoming a 'jogger'-maybe not a runner as such but definitely a jogger. I never really understood the difference, but presumable it refers to speed. Manie was a seasoned runner and would join us as we pounded the pavements, needing only a slight change of hand pressure on his elbow to guide him and run safely without falling. The man was an absolute inspiration and no doubt was the main reason I tried not to complain about the pain I was enduring during our runs.

Reaching the one mile mark was a great achievement, but Manie insisted that we aim for 5miles. This seemed like a bit over the top but then why not try. I had no idea how long this would take. In fact I don't actually remember how long it took to reach the goal, but reach it we did. Claude had decided by this stage to throw in the towel which was fair enough as he had a problem with one leg, having suffered from infantile paralysis (polio) as a child. His efforts were amazing and I admire Claud for his unending tenacity. He retains this quality till today living in the southern part of Israel.

We met a true inspiration in the person of Dennis Jones, who had run the 90 km long Comrades marathon, a gruelling race between Durban and Pietermaritzburg, alternating direction every year, a true challenge if ever there was one. Dennis joined us on an evening jog and we looked and listened to him extolling the virtues of the magical event. How was it possible to run such a distance, never mind the challenging terrain? The idea was incomprehensible.

Ronnie and I persisted with our 5 milers, till one day Ronnie suggested we should try and run 10 miles (16 km). Surely this was to be the final challenge? Where would we choose a route to run? It so happens that on the East Rand where we lived in Benoni, the next town to us was called Springs, exactly 16 km away from the border of Benoni. This surely was to be the route as it was virtually flat all the way without any challenging hills.

Late one Saturday afternoon we were dropped off in Springs, wearing our tracksuits and tennis shoes, our wives waving us goodbye and wishing us luck. I've no doubt that they thought we were mad. We set off with light fading rather rapidly and storm clouds suddenly making an appearance overhead. Then the heavens opened up and drenched us totally. It was difficult to differentiate between road and pavement as both were under water. It was only the lights of oncoming traffic that illuminated our surroundings, each passing car and truck drenching us even further. The crutch of my tracksuit pants was full of water and hanging at the level of my knees. What a nightmare the run turned out to be. On the positive side we had no time to be considering feeling tired or thirsty, survival was all we thought of. Not having any idea of the time, we battled on our epic journey. Suddenly a car approached us and stopped. It was our wives who were concerned about our welfare. They asked us to abort the run and get into the car. We declined. At this stage, giving up after so much effort was tantamount to being 'wimps', a term not yet discovered back then to describe losers. The rain started to subside when we made our triumphant entry to home, feeling elated and expecting to be welcomed as heroes, but that was not how the story ended. Both our wives were irate for having to be dragged out in wretched weather despite displaying concern. However they had the good grace to prepare some delicious soup, a welcoming sight indeed. A night to remember when we broke the 10 mile barrier.

A WEIGHTY PROBLEM

With all our endeavours and having overcome anterior knee pain, foot blisters and the likes, I was aware of a real change in my body weight. Within a relatively short time, my weight had dropped from 92 kg to a respectable 80 kg, a whopping 12 kg. The reason for this was two fold I reasoned. It was due to the running as well as drastically cutting down what I was stuffing into my mouth surely. This was a concerted effort for sure, something I had never thought of doing prior to this, as it was never necessary or so I thought. I was to discover to my detriment the following, namely:

LESSON 2: after the age of 25 things
are never going to be the same!

I would say the majority of the weight I lost occurred within a 16 week period. It really became effortless to my surprise and I ceased to try and lose any more In fact I stopped thinking about my neighbours comments although I never forgot them, what a nasty lady!

I managed to run at least three times a week, hardly ever changing the routine, always aiming for 10 km in the evening. Some of the runs I would meet Ronnie half way, but more often than not I ran alone. It wasn't always easy to meet the challenge as my workload in practice was heavy, added to which I had embarked upon another serious challenge and that was to attempt part one of the exam to become anaesthetist all by myself, something not to be taken lightly. This I might add is not how most people attempt the exam, rather choosing to do it in a teaching hospital. I was trying to fit everything into an already crowded schedule, which was not a good idea, as something was bound to give. I was biting off more than I could chew and I knew it.

I started missing a few runs trying to balance my life especially when I realised how demanding studying for the specialist exam actually was. My wife gently asked me one day if I had given up running which prompted me to get back into it more seriously.

Ronnie phoned me asking if I would like to join him in running the Springs Striders 20 miler(32km),being run in a few weeks. Suddenly the challenge was on and the butterflies in the stomach feeling was present. We had never run anything as long and had no idea how to approach it. We naively reasoned that we needed to be able to run 20 miles in preparation to be able to run 20 miles. Nothing, we later learnt, could be further from the truth.

We set out planning to reach a 20 mile distance in the week before the race almost reaching the goal but falling short by a half mile or so. The day arrived and we found ourselves nervously mingling with 250 runners of all shapes and sizes. It was my first exposure to so many runners none of whom we knew. I shall always remember the ubiquitous smell of 'wintergreen' liniment, rubbed into sore muscles not yet recovered from the last run. I was offered some and accepted. I had never actually used it but was willing to try as the liniment has a pleasant aroma. However I learnt a lesson that day regarding wintergreen and that was:

LESSON 3: always wash your hands after applying Wintergreen before going anywhere near your scrotum!

The stuff burns like hell when coming into contact with mucous membranes or eyes. It is the sort of mistake you only make once in a life time.

My recall of the race is limited and I don't remember my time or actual finishing position, but I was near the back of the field. There were a few stragglers left on the field. Ronnie had a better race than I had, we drove home feeling very tired but elated. I thought that I had reached my goal finally, namely I had managed to run a decent distance and had lost a fair amount of weight. There was no need to persist any longer reaching for greater heights. With a serious anaesthetic examination looming and no intention of ever running a marathon, at least at this stage of my life, I decided to put running temporarily on the back burner. This was not how things would turn out and I could never have predicted at this stage what the future held in store regarding my running career.

MOVING ON AFTER PASSING THE PRIMARY ANAESTHETIC EXAMINATION

It was my intention to complete my specialisation as an anaesthetist in Cape Town at the famous Groote Schuur Hospital where Christiaan Barnard performed the first heart transplant, but I had one more challenge offered to me by Ronnie before leaving for Cape Town. Ronnie was turning out to be real 'Iron Man'. I had to accept the challenge which was to run the Peter Korkie memorial 56 km ultra marathon between Pretoria and Germiston. Bear in mind I had not yet attempted a standard 42 km marathon, 32 km was the furthest I had run and not very well either. Nevertheless, I decided to take the challenge, only this time I would have to train on my own, which is character building to say the least. It would entail driving to Pretoria and leaving my car there, setting off accompanied by a patient of mine on his bicycle. He was an immigrant to South Africa, and had represented England in cycling at the Olympics previously. The reason for this arrangement was that my wife had refused to be involved as she though the idea insane. I should have read the danger signs earlier!

The day dawned for my practice run and off we set

for Pretoria early one Sunday morning whilst most were sleeping. I had no idea how much fluid I should carry as in the early seventies,the book on fluids had not yet been written. Initially there is a long hill which after a few kilometres levels out into a non ending continuation of undulations, too many to count. As the sun rose, the day turned from pleasantly cool to unpleasantly hot and I was starting to feel decidedly uncomfortable to put it mildly. I was getting very thirsty, my tongue sticking to my palate, which I knew meant for certain I was falling behind with my fluids. The trouble was we were miles from home and there were no farms or dwelling for several miles to come. I had no hat to shield my head, my shoulders were sore, my legs were cramping almost continuously and I had a royal headache, something I rarely experienced. In runners terms I was buggered! My cyclist pal was not doing too well either so I sent him home to recover. I would have to find help on my own. This was long before cell phones were even heard of.

I hobbled into a cafeteria in Atlasville on the outskirts of Benoni and pleaded with the owner to let me call my wife to come and collect me. My joy was short lived when my irate wife scolded me for being such an idiot and refused to collect me. I was shattered. I felt as if I could die any moment. I requested one more phone call which was to my friend and saviour, Rod Lagesen, who lived in our complex. Without hesitation he was over like a flash to save me. I could barely get into his Beetle without going into excruciating spasms. It was terrible. I felt awful. Helping me to get up the stairs in our apartment was trying, eventually Rod filled the bath with warm water, helped me to undress and eased me into the soothing water. Any thought of ever running the "Korkie" marathon were immediately banished. At that very moment I recall thinking that my running days were over for sure. I knew if I persisted my wife would never talk to me again but worse still just feeling so bad, I decided I never want to relive another moment like this.

Slightly more mobile after my hot bath but still in pain and nauseous, I slowly got into bed after some hot soup. I fell soundly asleep and slept several hours. When I awoke, the pain and nausea had passed and what woke me was a full bladder, a good sign that my kidneys were functioning for which I was extremely grateful. The next morning I had to be at work as usual. The negative feelings about running had disappeared like the morning dew and the race was on again. My wife had not spoken to me by the time I left for work.

I had learned several lessons that day, but if the truth be told, I would later on repeat a few errors several times not endearing myself to my 'better half'. It is said we are pigs for punishment, I know that is one of my serious shortcomings in life.

An interesting anecdote regarding my pulse rate. During my teens and especially at university, my resting pulse rate hovered around 55 beats/minute. With all the training I had done during my time in Benoni, my pulse rate dropped to 46/min and stand on my head, I could not get it to go any lower. Benoni is situated on the East rand near Johannesburg at an altitude or elevation of 1,646 meters / 5,400ft. above sea level.

Running or at least training at altitude for at least three weeks increases the levels of an enzyme 2,3,DPG which helps to increase the amount of oxygen available to the tissues. The less 2,3,DPG the less oxygen is given off from the haemoglobin molecule whose function it is to carry oxygen. So despite my efforts I was not going to benefit from altitude training to get my resting pulse rate down any lower. I would have to do something else if it were to come down at all.

I was very interested in physiology and cardiovascular physiology in particular. Remember I had just passed the primary exam in anaesthesia and physiology was the holy grail. We needed to understand it extremely well, and in an applied way. The buck stops with us anaesthetists after all. The problem though is that physiological changes in endurance sport are not seen in 'normal' people who lead sedentary lives. The text books tend to describe normal people who on average have resting pulse rates around 72beats / minutes. That would be considered abnormal in a long distance marathon runner.

Glancing at AP(anterior/posterior) chest x-rays of weight lifters and distance runners, one can often see cardiac enlargement which can be difficult to differentiate from cardiac enlargement seen in hypertension and other pathological causes. It becomes obvious at post mortem when dissecting the heart that the difference in wall thickness in the three mentioned groups becomes apparent. In the runner the dilated heart is mainly due to enlargement of the chambers while the ventricular myocardium thickness remains relatively normal, whereas the weight lifter has a smaller volume ventricle with a thickened myocardium, due to the increased resistance offered to the heart during systole or contraction of the heart. It should be stated that the enlarged cardiac dimensions in both groups of sportspersons is regarded as abnormal in that they differ from the norm. Whether changes in the runner's dilated heart are as serious as those in the weight lifter, I think is debatable. I like to think not, based on the following:

The muscle of the heart receives oxygen and nutrients during the rest phase of the cardiac cycle, so called diastole which is the period when the left ventricle is relaxing after ejecting blood into the aorta. The aortic valve which separates the left ventricle from the cavity of the aorta snaps closed, allowing the internal pressure in the ventricle to fall rapidly while the pressure in the aorta remains high as blood is propelled forward, aided by the elastic recoil of the healthy aortic wall as well as closure of the aortic valve. This enables the pressure gradient between the empty left ventricle and the high pressure in the aorta, to fill the coronary vessels and thus in turn allowing the myocardium to receive oxygen and nutrients. It stands to reason that the slower the heart rate, the longer will be the rest period leading to better filling. The thinner the myocardium, the less mass of muscle has to be supplied and therefore the less the demand for oxygen.

It can therefore be gathered from this simplistic explanation, that the work of the heart is less when a large amount of blood is pumped slowly compared to a smaller volume being pumped at a faster rate.

The Peter Korkie came and went and compared to my first 32 km race in Springs, the Korkie was much better, with insignificant pain during and after but all in all it was a reasonable race. Again I have no recall of my time. The year was 1974 and I would soon be heading down to Cape Town to complete my studies in anaesthesia at Groote Schuur hospital (GSH-or fondly known by one and all as 'Grotties')

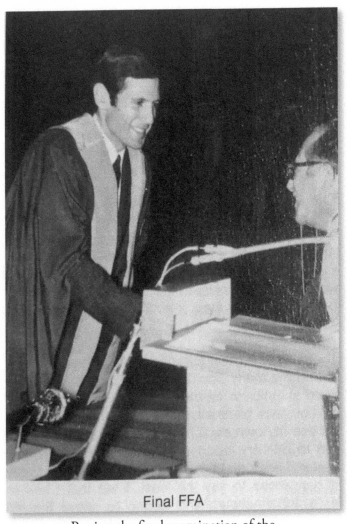

Final FFA

Passing the final examination of the
Fellowship of Anaesthetics of the College
of Medicine of South Africa (1977)

TIME ON MY HANDS

For the first time in years I was able to relax somewhat, due to my new rosters and time tables in my designation as a new registrar in the department of anaesthetics being far less demanding than my life as a general practitioner in Benoni. This luxurious situation was due to the fact that I had passed the primary exam, the first hurdle whilst in practice. I was only able to have a crack at the final exam once two years had passed and having shown adequate competence in my new speciality, something I would be judged on by my professors and senior consultants.

All this meant that I would be able to spend more time running in my new environment which I would learn to relish. Cape Town would prove to be a runners delight, with unmatched scenery and beauty, not to mention adequate hills and even a mountain in the centre of the city to really challenge me to literally reach new heights with my love of running.

Being registered with the University of Cape Town as part of my obligations in studying at GSH, I was entitled to join the varsity running club. This was to be a major step in my improvement as a runner. Most of the members were somewhat younger than me. As students they were involved in a first degree whereas I had 5 years as a general practitioner over them. I realised early that I needed to put in a lot of work to keep up with the pack on our training runs which included 8 km time trials in Newlands forest, a beautiful forest on the slopes of Table Mountain. On the weekends, we would often increase the distance gradually to 16-20 km with runs down to Hout Bay, ending with a swim in the cold Atlantic waters.

There were some seriously good runners in the club, one of whom was Dave Levick, who had recently broken the record for the 90 km Comrades Marathon by far. Dave gave a new meaning to training which rubbed off onto us all. Another future bright star was a recently qualified young doctor Tim Noakes, who would establish himself as a sports medicine professor at UCT and world authority, leading to research in many aspects of sport, in particular long distance running. Training methodology, fluid intake and many other subjects would be experimented with and undergo radical change, some tried and tested concepts challenged and accepted by most, but others remaining to this day to be controversial and as yet unsettled.

Added to this, nutrition in sport and in general started to enter into the ever changing picture, nutrition definitely being controversial and certainly not all theories universally accepted. I refer to concepts such as intermittent fasting, the Keto diet, low carbohydrate and high fat diets . I will allude to this in detail in part two of the book.

In 1975 when I moved to Cape Town to embark on my new carrier, the accepted method for preparing for a race was known as carbohydrate loading or commonly

"Carbo-Loading," the so-called Saltin diet, named after the Swedish physiologist Bengt Saltin.

The full pre race diet started six days prior to the race avoiding any form of carbohydrate for three days, only eating protein while exercising in an effort to deplete the muscle and liver glycogen stores, the idea being, that the three days prior to the race would revert to only eating carbohydrates in order to 'supercharge' the body's glycogen stores before the race.

I personally only once ever tried the full six day diet, but found it far too strenuous. On the evening of the third carbohydrate free diet, I could barely crawl home, being hypoglycaemic, acidotic and extremely weak. I managed to run a hot bath after gorging my way through anything I could find in the kitchen cupboard. I could have eaten the plate I was so depleted.

LESSON 4: never gorge yourself after severe carbohydrate depletion!

Immediately after my despicable act of gluttony, I developed acute gastric dilatation, something to be avoided. It is very dangerous and must be avoided at all costs. I had splinting of my diaphragm and at best could only breathe with rapid and shallow breaths. Picture me on all fours in a hot tub gasping for breath. I was not sure that this wasn't going to end badly. Panic was about to set in when the symptoms slowly began to subside. I was able to breathe more freely after about 20 minutes. I managed to extricate myself from the bath without my family being any the wiser thank goodness. I can't imagine the repercussions from my wife who had already reacted negatively to one of my running escapades back when I was a general practitioner.

I finally accepted that a modified form of the Saltin diet suited me, namely Carbohydrate loading for three days prior to the race. This seemed to be adopted by most runners at the time and served its purpose just fine. Fluid intake on the other hand was not properly worked out in the mid 70's by any means and we went through many regimes till we settled on one that seemed reasonable.

My first year in Cape town was 1975, and I was to discover a new level of running, thanks to being able to train with the likes of excellent runners at UCT. More important though was the fact that there was no shortage of hills and even Table Mountain to run up. Initially it was challenging but after a while I started relishing the steep gradients and realise their importance in getting fit.

I had not yet run a standard marathon by the time the famous Two Oceans marathon came about, run on the Easter weekend. My first Two Oceans was a memorable one, finding the magnificent views a pleasant distraction from the discomfort experienced after the 28 km mark when tiredness started to set in as we approached the Chapmans Peak climb. I was surrounded by friends who's banter also helped to dissipate the discomfort. All in all the race was good, not having aspired to anything other than just to complete the race in one piece.

The next year I was keen to line up once more on the Villagers sports field, a lot fitter and more of a runner than simply a 'jogger'. By this stage, after having trained a lot harder than initially in Benoni, my resting pulse rate had come down to about 38/min, something I could not achieve prior to coming to Cape Town. The race was run in the rain for most of the way which I found enjoyable. I bettered my time from the previous year by half an hour which was encouraging, finishing in 5 hours. The gun was fired at 6 hours being the cut off point for the56 km ultra marathon.

At prize giving out on the rugby field, we were sitting around in groups with our families where I noticed a straggler coming in who seemed to be in a bad way. I took him and lay him down in the shade of a car, realising that he was clinically severely dehydrated. I had a litre of saline in the boot of my car, and gave it to him intravenously. He perked up soon after. I realised that something needed to be done to prevent this sort of thing happening with an ultra marathon like the 56 km Two Oceans. I approached Chet Sainsbury, the race organiser and explained the situation, so Chet appointed me as the doctor in charge of medical tent which was established the next year.

MY FIRST COMRADES MARATHON 1975

Having completed the Two Oceans marathon, I had still not run a standard 42 km marathon. If I wanted to run the 90 km Comrades marathon between Durban and Pietermaritzburg in Natal, I would need to submit a time for the marathon in order to qualify for the race as there was a cut off point of 1500 runners. Hugh Amore, the UCT running club captain therefore organised a run of 42 km, so that those wanting to qualify could do so. My time was 3 hours 38 min.

This race was going to be the biggest running challenge to date for a few reasons and was to be a watershed event in my running career. I was to meet up with my old friend Ronnie from Benoni and his cousin Harry would 'second' us both on the run, something that would turn out to be disastrous. In these early days of the Comrades marathon, traffic was allowed on the road. The race itself was held on the old road between Durban and Pietermaritzburg and was unable to handle heavy traffic which there inevitable was on race day. In short, I saw Harry once in the beginning of the race and never again till the finish as Ronnie and I separated early on in the race due the traffic chaos. I had to run the race with virtually not having any fluid intake, save for a few gulps from onlookers who gave me what they could. I hobbled into Pietermaritzburg late that afternoon, ten and a half hours after setting off from Durban, cramping severely even as I tried to mount the pavement. It was terrible. Realising that I was in trouble and could easily go into renal failure, I hastily took myself off to a nearly clinic and gave myself 2.5 lites of balanced salt solution Intra venously. I soon had a diuresis and vowed that that would never happen again.

LESSON 5: Never allow yourself to get into severe fluid deficit!

Following this near catastrophe, I became acutely aware of fluid intake and started experimenting with various volumes.

In 1977, I successfully passed my final examination of the college of Medicine of South Africa, becoming an anaesthetist. I would still need time at the teaching hospital before being able to register as a consultant, and this would be perfect in allowing me the time to train more.

I took a month off in May to do a GP locum in the Transkei as I needed to boost my miserable salary at the hospital. Besides I enjoy the sort of medicine one gets to practice in the rural areas of Africa. The pathology is always advanced and most times obvious, with only really ill patients presenting at the surgery. The conditions most commonly seen were Tuberculosis including constrictive pericarditis, something rarely seen in the first world. Avitaminosis, gastroenteritis, measles, malnutrition in children, both Kwashiorkor (protein shortage) and Marasmus, which is insufficient intake of all nutrition. Trauma from accidents and violence, and pregnancy which needed careful assessment as far as gestation was concerned, as the outcome could mean the difference between life and death for some unsuspecting bloke. Remember, most of the menfolk of the Transkei worked away from home for long periods of time on the gold mines.

I had promised my dear friend Tim Farquharson, that I would run the Comrades with him in 1977, but didn't take into consideration that I would be in the Transkei during the month running up to the marathon. Nevertheless, we ran it very conservatively and Tim was happy with the result. Shortly after this, Tim emigrated to Aukland, New Zealand where he practiced as a successful GP.

BREAKING THE THREE HOUR BARRIER

Training in 1978 was to take on a new meaning. Not only was I going to step up quality but also quantity. Percy Cerutty, the eccentric Australian athletics coach inspired us to new heights. I recall a statement of his which stuck in my mind-"If you want to run fast, you need to move your legs faster and take bigger steps". It sounded reasonable but how to achieve this?

We started training everyday, seldom resting unless one felt jaded. We often ran three times a day which was in retrospect unwise, but it did lead to a rapid improvement in levels of fitness. However it also lead to illness and injury, with bronchitis often a precursor to other injuries, like tendonitis, ITB injuries (Iliotibial band), bursitis, and many others. Foolishly we thought that we could 'run through' these injuries. Missing a day of training was unacceptable and without realising it, we were making a fetish of running. It became all consuming and in fact addictive. It would take many years to actually realise the possible damage this excessive training program would cause to my heart, but if the truth be told, I would not have believed it, after all, how could being so fit do harm to oneself when I had never felt better?

On some days we would run three times. One could expect to do 8 to 10 km in the early morning, followed by hill springs or track work in the afternoon to build speed. Finally at the end of the day we would end with a gentle 10 to 16 km.

Hill springs entailed sprinting flat out up a steep gradient for about 150 meters, lifting knees and pumping arms. We would do a set of ten which was more than enough.

Watching my diet carefully and keeping calorie intake as low as possible the weight simply fell away. I went down to 76 kg, and looked decidedly skeletal. Despite this I was feeling wonderful. Without realising that I was heading toward anorexia, I continued to train hard. A few warnings signs should have made me wisen up. People told me I was looking gaunt and I loved it. Some said I was looking better and it signalled that I wasn't training enough.

I needed very little sleep and in fact often found it difficult to sleep. After a night on call at the hospital without any sleep I often got home, put on running shoes and headed for the hills. This was madness, but I was loving it. I never felt tired whatsoever.

My claim to fame, which my son Graeme still to this day uses as my yardstick, is that I could hold my breath for 30 seconds while running up Table Mountain. Only a madman would contemplate doing this!

The Peninsula marathon in 1978, from Cape Town foreshore to Simonstown, was to be the race I would try and break the 3 hour barrier. I would have to improve my one and only marathon time at this stage by 38 minutes, a tall order I thought. The race was well planed and I ran a disciplined race at around 4 minutes and 10 seconds a kilometre. I ended up doing 2 hours 52 minutes which would turn out to be my fasted standard marathon going forward.

I realised however that my strength lay not in speed per se, as although my time was respectable, it certainly wasn't great. I soon realised where my strength lay and that was I was able to sustain that speed for longer than my pals were able to do. I was also able to run up steep gradients faster and for longer than all my pals. This was baffling even to Tim Noakes. Could I possible get a silver medal in the Two Oceans marathon? It would mean I had to be able to run the 56 km in under 4 hours which was a formidable task indeed.

Statistically it was claimed that to be able to do this, one needed to have a marathon time of 2:36, much faster than my 2:52. It meant I would have to run my fasted marathon time of 2:52 up to the marathon mark, remembering that this, unlike the Peninsular marathon, was not flat, but traversed serious hills all the way. Then from the marathon mark I would have to run the next 4 gruelling kilometres at a reduced rate of 5 minutes a kilometre uphill till we reached Constantia neck. This left the last 10 kilometres to be run at slightly faster than 4:10/km, a tall order for any reasonable runner.

Statistically no more than 10% of the field qualifies for a silver medal. Was I up to the challenge? I certainly was going to attack it seriously. One thing I had learned was that commitment to take on a challenge was all important if one was to succeed. I had a few real challenges in my life to date. Getting into first year medical school was one of them, getting into second year even more of a challenge. Passing the primary anaesthetic exam from general practice without any help in the form of lectures was even more difficult, but I decided I wanted these goals badly.

My motto at the time was —

Nail my scrotum to the chair and don't get up till I know the work !

It worked a charm.

Race day arrived and I was up for the challenge. One always has the jitters before a race but this one even more so. I hardly slept at all on the night before the race, but wasn't too concerned about this. I had slept well two nights before the race, which was deemed to be adequate.

I lined up near the front of the pack, something I was loathe to do but here I has no choice as after the gun went off, there was a mad dash to squeeze through the wide gate leading off the field onto the road. I had to avoid the bottle neck if I stood any chance of sticking to the planned 4:10 /km.

Having made it through the gate my heart was racing and I was breathing fiercely. It took a good two kilometres to settle down to my pace. It is never a good idea to exceed one's desired speed, as there is always a price to pay sooner or later.

My seconds for the race were two other members from the anaesthetic department. Chris Swart was riding his 250cc Honda and Michael de Haan, was on the pillion, facing backwards, ready to call out my time after each kilometre. I needed to strictly adhere to the plan if I was to succeed. Amazingly enough, I managed to stick very closely to the time and I felt good.

They got me through to the marathon mark in 2:52, which was remarkable. I was now allowed the luxury of slowing down to 5 min/km, but considering the steep gradient up to the top, even 5 min/km was fast. On the way up to Constantia neck, the Hout Bay cemetery lies on the right side of the road. Passing it on this occasion brought a smile to my face. I thought of the inscription on one of the grave stones, in a prominent position which said-

"And God saw that you were weary and called you to rest"

Hopefully I would last a little longer!

The last 10 kilometres down from the neck were mostly downhill, except for two nasty hills, named fuck-it no.1 and fuck-it no.2, both which were gut wrenching inclines. I was doing my best despite feeling sore and looking for reason to stop which I knew I would never do. My mind was crowded with all sorts of thoughts, some positive, others negative. It was a mind game all the way. My body was aching but that I could deal with. It is amazing what punishment we put ourselves through, only to achieve a goal which in years to come, nobody other one self and a few friends remember. The medals lose their shine, tucked away in some bottom draw maybe never to be seen again other than in some pawnshop by some stranger, completely oblivious of how they were achieved in the first place.

I crossed the line in 3 hrs and 55 minutes, and achieved my goal. I was ecstatic. I couldn't wipe the smile of my face.

Could I possibly achieve a silver in Comrades?

So far the year 1978 was turning out to be memorable, with a 2:52 in the Peninsula marathon, a 3:55 in the Two Oceans. Winning a silver in the 90 km ultra marathon to be run at the end of May would mean running under seven and a half hours, or in other words at 5 minutes per kilometre, a mere doddle compared to the 4:10min/km in the Two Oceans. However there is a difference between 56 km and 90 km. According to most achieving a silver in the Two Oceans was more difficult than in the Comrades. Time would tell.

It was said then that one needed at least three months to recover from a standard 42 km marathon before contemplating another. This was fine in theory, but the marathon season in South Africa was structured in such a way, not allowing enough recovery time if one wanted to attempt all the classic races. Nobody calling himself a runner would not consider doing them all regardless. The Comrades took a severe toll on the body and any sensible person was supposed to rest for a year before attempting any competition. Jogging per se was fine but serious training not advised. I don't recall any of my friends ever heeding the advice which is why most of us at one time or another, nursed injuries throughout our running careers. The fallout from these excesses would manifest after many years. The reason we were oblivious to any possible cardiovascular damage following ultra distance training was that not enough time had passed for this damage to develop. The sport was not wildly popular then. It would take another 30 plus years to start seeing the fallout from the long distance running, and even then it was not universally accepted that this 'over training' indeed was the cause for ubiquitous cardiac lesions which started appearing in well trained athletes across the board. We forget that Pheidippides was the first person to run the distance circa 490 BC and died as a result of exhaustion. Maybe we should have paid more attention to this event.

Training for the 90 km race meant aiming for at least 100 km per week. The plan was to run a long one on the weekends such as a neck to neck, starting at and ending at Constantia neck, a mere 50 km run covering plenty of hills. Mondays would be a slowish 16 km run and most other days either once or twice a day, 8 or 10 km, making sure we ended with at least 100 km for the week.

Errol, a neurosurgeon from Natal, launched himself from nowhere, to end 4th in the Comrades, boasting that his secret was to run 200 km /week for several weeks prior to the race. This suddenly caused everyone to jack up their milage. I tried on one occasion to do this but failed dismally, only reaching 160 km for the week. I was dejected. In reality there were few if any who could match this training program. Sadly it worked only once for Errol, and he developed a serious running injury, dehiscence of the pubic symphysis, forcing him to give up on what was a promising career.

I made sure at this stage to mix my training between speed, hill climbing strength and long endurance, hoping to avoid any injury along the way if possible.

I would like to mention that I had become aware of palpitations from time to time but disregarded them as innocent skipped or extra beats, usually very short lived. I put it down to the fact that my resting pulse was 32 beats/ min of which I was particularly proud. This surely was the reason for my palpitations. If the normal SA (Sino-Atrial node) heart rate was 70 beats/minute, and the AV (Atrioventricular) nodal rate was set at around 45/minute as a safety net, then my slow rate of 32 beats /minute was surely causing the variety of arrhythmias I was experiencing.

In theatre one day a few weeks before the big day, I was administering anaesthesia to a patient when I experienced a few beats in a row. I put ECG leads on myself and recorded several short runs of unifocal ventricular extrasystoles, a first for me. I sat up surprised but not yet really concerned as they did not fulfil the requirements for treating, such as longer than 5 in a row or multifocal etc. They subsided after a few deep inhalations and I continued with the anaesthetic.

On the next Saturday, the week prior to the Comrades, the running club organised a fast 16 km race inclusive of hills and flats, which was to be our last training session prior to race day. I was feeling fine and set off at pace. About half way through I started to feel runs of palpitations but it wasn't too perturbed about them. My breathing was fine and I felt nothing untoward. I was just concerned as to why I was getting them. I finished the 16 kms and other than a slight pull in a calf muscle which was successfully cross-frictioned away (using the Maitland technique), I was fine. I put it down to a combination of tiredness and excessive training. I needed to take it easy before the race. All that was left was to carbohydrate load for three days.

The big day arrived and I joined the thousands of other runners outside the Pietermaritzburg City hall huddled together in the early morning cold, the smell of wintergreen mentholated rub highly noticeable and the loudspeakers blaring out the by now the irritating "Chariots of Fire" anthem, ubiquitous at all running events. Initially it was stirring and fired up the spirit to do one's best but it had been played to death at every race. It was exciting all the same and I was enthralled by it all. I never stopped being a child and have made it my goal never to grow up, as being a kid is so much more fun.

I ran the race in the company of Tim Noakes and a young Irish lass, Isavel Roche-Kelly, a student at the University of Cape Town, who held the ladies record for the race. She was the first woman to achieve a silver medal in the Comrades marathon. Isavel was slight of build and ran hardly breaking into a sweat, while we males clearly didn't handle our fluid loss as efficiently as women it seemed. Tragically Isavel was killed while cycling back in Ireland a few year later, a sad loss indeed.

The race was memorable for a few reasons. The crowds lined the road for virtually the whole distance, spurring the runners on regardless of where they came from. Some went to great lengths to set up stands giving away drinks and all sorts of fun stuff creating a real carnival atmosphere. However there comes a time in the race for some runners sooner than later, that we stop seeing the funny side and start to get irritable instead at some of these antics. One such incident I shan't forget running down the long Field's hill approach into Pine Town. A fellow and his girlfriend or wife, parked a four poster brass bed on the side of the road, lying on the bed between soft silk sheets sipping champagne and shouting out-"Keep it up old chap, not far to go" In retrospect it was funny but at the time they were lucky I didn't jump into the bed and clobber them.

Having reached the 45th cutting, several kilometres outside of Durban, I was feeling decidedly under the weather. My shoulders and back were sore, my legs were aching but fortunately not cramping. My entire body was begging me to stop. In short, I was wrecked! At this stage I could have rested for an hour and still finished the race, but that was not the plan. After all I had been through in training and having experienced the wrath of my wife who had to endure my extreme running antics, and warned me not to come home without a silver medal, stopping was not an option. I truly felt that I could die any moment I felt so awful.

Reaching the top of the Berea, a mere 4 kilometres from Kingsmead stadium, the finish of the race, I came upon a fellow runner, Angus from Cape Town, lying on the pavement refusing to budge another step. His seconders were shouting expletives at him, to get up and finish the race. I knew exactly what he was feeling. The downhill to the stadium required a supreme effort despite the gradient. The noise from the waiting crowds was electrifying. Suddenly the strength needed to finished came from deep within. I wasn't sure exactly of the time, but I knew if I didn't stop, I could make the cut off. As I crossed the line I looked up and saw the time - 7 hours 26 minutes. I had achieved the impossible. The silver was in the bag. Seconds before the 7:30 cut off time Angus collapsed over the line also finishing with his silver. What a day!

The elation of my silver medal was indescribable. Never in my wildest dreams during my early running days in Benoni as a GP, could I imagine getting a sliver medal, let alone just completing the Comrades.

The elation lasted a short while as I needed to fly home to Cape Town from Durban across the southern part of South Africa. At the airport it wasn't difficult to see who had run the race. Those climbing up the stairs backwards to board the plain definitely ran the race. Seeing so many doing it brought a smile to my face. I was hurting but I wasn't going to be seen doing the same thing. What followed during the recovery phase was extremely trying to say the least. My body was depleted and I was in no shape to even consider running anytime soon. I remained relatively tachycardic, my resting pulse was around 65 beats/minute, a far cry from my usual 32beats/minute, indicating that my body was not back to a pH of 7.4 yet. My acid base balance system was working overtime to return me back to normal biochemical values.

My legs were taking a long time to get back to normal. For two months after the race I wasn't able to sit down slowly on the toilet seat. I simply had to flop down onto the seat. Getting up was fine but sitting down was another matter. I had clearly overdone it but at least had a silver medal to show for my troubles.

The 24 hour challenge

June and July are the winter months in the Cape and winters as a rule are relatively mild. It is also the rainy season, not exactly conducive to outdoor running. Then after the break once more the marathons start coming around again and there are several to choose from in the Cape, all of which take place in beautiful surroundings like the Cape winelands. In any year it is possible to run at least eight marathons in the Cape excluding the two ultra marathons. It was never my intention to run each one flat out but use them as training runs at best. Added to these were a host of half marathons which one could use as good training

I ran marathons whenever I felt like it, but made no

fetish of having to run each one. As far as I was concerned I had reached all my running goals, namely a sub three hour standard marathon in the Peninsula marathon, silvers in both Comrades and Two oceans. The only challenge remaining was to see if I could repeat the silvers again. I knew that running under three hours for the marathon was not a challenge anymore.

Every year the running association organised a 24 hour challenge, requiring six members in each team, to run a mile around the Green Point stadium track in 24 hours and see which team covered the most distance. The race began at 1700 hours on a Friday evening and continued for 24 hrs.

This proved to be a daunting challenge as I was on call on the Thursday night which gave me little opportunity for sleep unfortunately. This meant I would go without sleep for two nights in a row, not a good idea. Besides me running, I was to be doctor for two other members of our running club, namely VOB or varsity old boys club. I was no longer a registered member of UCT so was no longer able to run in UCT colours. The two were Bruce Matthews and Graham Dacomb. They were going for the two man record which even I thought was madness. I had to give both of them IV fluids on two occasions during the night besides my own running, which proved rather tricky time wise.

At the end of the race I was shattered and slept solidly till Sunday morning. I woke up with palpitations and 'cannon wave' pulsations in my neck, a very uncomfortable feeling indeed, which lasted more or less intermittently all day. I went to work on Monday with these waves pounding in my neck, so after the list I lay down and took my own ECG. What I saw alarmed me no end. I was experiencing runs of unifocal ventricular extrasystoles which wasn't the main worry, I saw non concordant T-waves in AVF which I'd never seen before. Could this be a Myocardial infarct?

My heart sank as I drove home to show my ECG to my neighbour Brian, a brilliant physician who was also a qualified radiologist. He too was uncertain and suggested I see the professor of cardiology, Wally Beck. Wally arranged for me to have an echocardiogram of the heart, as he thought it could possibly be HOCM, or hypertrophic obstructive cardiomyopathy, which is not news I wanted to hear. Luckily, the consensus of opinion of all the senior members of the department was that I didn't have either HOCM or an MI. Apparently my picture was similar to the Bushmen of the Kalahari and the African miners toiling away at great depths in SA's gold mines. To say I was relieved was an understatement. I would live to run another day!

Working in private anaesthetic practice and being on the staff of Groote Schuur Hospital part time, my teaching hospital, afforded me time to run, but it was becoming difficult to fit in long runs and lead a normal life with the family.

We reached a stage where my wife gave me an ultimatum regarding the long weekend runs. If I wanted to do a long run on the weekend, it would have to be in my own time and had to be over by the time she woke up on Sunday morning, so that we could spend the day together as a family. Fair enough I thought but fitting in a long run was going to be tricky.

The problem was solved in a very unusual way. Bruce Mathews, Graeme Lindenberg and I would set off at 02:30 on Sunday morning and run from my home to Cape Point nature reserve and then on to Noordhoek, a run of 65 km. Watering points were petrol stations as no cafes were open at this unearthly hour and we carried whatever nourishment we thought we needed. Dawn broke only by the time we were in the Cape Point nature reserve, darkness giving way to a magical African sunrise, seen only by those who venture our at the crack of dawn.

Margie, Bruce's dedicated wife was the only one who would consider picking us from the end point. I shall never forget her kindness. I would get home just before the family was stirring and would shower, in order to be ready for a busy day with the family. I dared not mention being tired, this would have caused unhappiness, and despite just about falling asleep standing, I complied with the agreement. This continued for a few months prior to my last of seven Comrades runs. It was unsustainable and I was no longer enamoured by the idea of running any more Comrades marathons. I had achieved three silver Comrade medals and four bronze medals and I was not interested in running 10 to qualify for a permanent number.

The Two Oceans was different. Here I was part of the race already, having established the medical tent which was working well by any standards. Besides, the race was run in my home town Cape Town which made it all the more attractive.

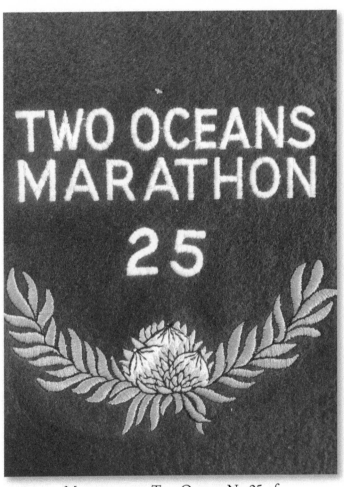

My permanent Two Oceans No.25 of
which I am very proud (1985)

Running my tenth Two Oceans Marathon

When I look back at the marathons I ran during my life time, I can say unequivocally that my best run was my tenth Two Oceans, the race where I would win my permanent race number, which is no. 25. This means I was the 25th person to have run ten Two Ocean marathons. Now there are thousands who have reached this mile stone. The number sits proudly framed on my book shelf where I can see it and reminisce over my glorious heydays of running.

My son Graeme, aged 12 years at the time, asked me if he could cycle next to me for the race. He needed to keep out of the way of runners, knowing just how irate we can get when pain and hunger and dehydration set in.

It was to be an auspicious occasion, and a bunch of my best pals, none of whom had managed to achieve a silver medal in the Two Oceans, asked me if I would act as pace setter for the race. I of course agreed. They knew the plan well but had never managed to stick with it. Could it be any different this time? The pace had to be 4:10/km to the marathon mark, then 5min/km up to Constantia neck, and then last ten kilometres-"balls to the wall"! There was to be no surging at any stage I demanded, as this generally would lead to an early demise. They all agreed.

This of course meant getting to the marathon mark in 2hours 52 minutes. Any thing slower would make getting a silver most unlikely. They all knew this. It was a big ask.

The weather for the race was perfect, a fine drizzle for the first half of the race. The race was going to plan until we reached Noordhoek Valley crossroads, where a very large crowd had gathered to cheer the runners on. The tendency to speed up usually occurs in situations like this and before I knew it, our group broke up and headed off much too fast, leaving me behind. I instinctively knew this was the end of the plan. I was amazed but more disappointed in the group.

I got to the half way mark of 28 kms at the start of Chapmans Peak which was no laughing matter. Hills were my forte so I was very comfortable going up but I had lost some time by the time I reached to top of Chapmans Peak. From the peak down to Hout Bay was all down hill, another dangerous place for surging. I had not yet met up with my pals who ran off leaving me behind. Maybe they were right and I was wrong all the time. On reaching Hout Bay where the road levels out and the climb to Constantia neck begins, I suddenly met up with the group, looking sorry for themselves. Not one was able to join my train to the end. In joggers terms they were 'buggered,' truly a sorry sight! I continued on to the marathon mark, Graeme on his bike never leaving my side, only to reach the mark in 3 hours exactly, a far cry from the 2:52 I need to get the silver. I had to make up 8 minutes which seemed an impossible task. I wasn't going to dwell on this going up the hill. I didn't ask for times, I pushed on as hard as I could. I reached the top feeling happy to be there but with no time to contemplate the niceties of life. Someone yelled to me that I had 40 minutes to do the last 10 kilometres in. This was unachievable as I had been running at best 4:10/km. I would have to run even faster.

I set off towards the finish striding it out, thinking of the permanent number I would love to get, rather than thinking of the silver medal. However I seemed to be running effortlessly till I reached the watering point set up by our running club. Friendly faces urged me on, but suddenly my wheels fell off just past the water station. Was I even going to finish? Miraculously the feeling was short lived and I perked up once again. Who knows what brought it on and more importantly how it managed to pass off.

The last 3 kilometres were hectic and Graeme was there urging me on. " You are going to make it dad-your'e almost there!" Finally the field was in sight, the noise was deafening. Graeme on his bike was not allowed onto the field and we parted ways after 56 km. I had 100 meters to the line and amazingly enough I was going to break 4 hours. My time was 3 hours, 59 minutes. I managed to run the last 10 kms in 39 minutes, something I had never dreamed of being able to do. I went on to run 17 Two Oceans marathons till I unfortunately got hepatitis-A, stopping me in my tracks and preventing me from running any more ultras. I ended with 3 silver medals in both the Comrades and Two Oceans marathon. I have no complaints.

Medical tent at the two Oceans marathon

My discovery of a dehydrated runner languishing in the hot sun after the 1976 Two Oceans, and subsequently resuscitating him, lead to the establishment of the medical tent for which I was given free rein to organise as I wished. The management instituted in the tent was based solely on clinical grounds, mainly from my experience as an anaesthetic registrar at the GSH teaching hospital. I might add here that at the same time I was commanding officer (Lt Col) of 20 field ambulance battalion, a citizen force non conventional unit established in the Cape, where additional experience was gained in treating dehydrated troops in the field. The African climate can be a cruel environment to operate in.

Dehydration is a clinical assessment based on a history of duration of fluid restriction or any abnormal loss such as diarrhoea and or vomiting. Added to this thirst, dryness of the mouth, loss of skin turgor, tachycardia and orthostatic hypotension (low blood pressure on standing), reduced jugular venous pressure (JVP), as well as reduced urine output. Insertion of a central catheter will shown a decrease in central venous pressure(CVP).

At the outset, we never intended measuring CVP in the medical tent, our assessment would be made purely on clinical grounds. We judged dehydration to be mild, moderate or severe. This rough scale would indicate losses from between 3litres (4%body weight) to 7litres (10% body weighting a 70 kg person). In a few seriously dehydrated runners decreased cognition was a clear indication of even greater losses. Two runners were brought in unconscious, with loss of the eyelash reflex, equitable with a state of anaesthesia.

I stress that we "eye-balled" the patients as they were brought in and according to their presenting symptoms, we would either treat by simply lying the patients down, with legs elevated and giving oral fluids until we had an improvement. Those displaying more severe symptoms were treated with a litre of balanced salt solution and waiting for a response this. If more was needed we would give a second litre. Often there was a good response after the second lite and on average we found that two litres sufficed. An interesting observation was seen in the majority of cases which was a sudden onset of severe cramping of the legs as the fluid infused the tissues. This cramping was short lived and was followed by an almost euphoric period with the cessation of the cramping.

By continual observation we decided on wether to continue IV fluids or not. Over the years in the tent, two litres was expected to resolve any serious issues resulting from inadequate intake during the race. The most we ever gave patients were 5 litres, but these were few and far between.

How much to drink during a race remained problematic for many years. In the late 70's we tried to quantify an amount but clearly this would not be able to suit all comers. For starters, females runners, who on average were lighter than the men seemed to handle fluid loss far better than the men. The range of fluid intake varied from 100 ml/Hr to 1000ml/Hr. Believe it or not some of us managed to drink a whopping litre every hour for a few marathons, but it quickly became evident that this was excessive. Running at speed with fluid sloshing around in one's stomach was most uncomfortable and clearly wrong.

It was after this period that Prof Noakes from the UCT sports foundation decided to initiate research into the problem of fluid intake and our Two Oceans tent was a good place to initiate this.

I was approached by Tim and agreed to allot a section to him and his team for the purposes of conducting research into why runners collapsed. I stress that this was done after runners had ceased trying to drink a litre every hour in races.

In 1991 Tim Noakes published a paper* (of which I was coauthor with Neil Berlinski, and Lindsay Weight) entitled

Collapsed Runners: Blood Biochemical Changes After IV Fluid Therapy. This appeared in the journal **The Physician and Sportsmedicine,** vol19.No 7,July 91.

In brief the article claimed that the effects of routine IV fluid therapy on blood biochemical values in collapsed runners have not been studied. We measured serum sodium concentrations and other indicators of fluid status in 32 collapsed and 16 non collapsed runners after the 56 km race. Twenty-six(31%) of the collapsed received IV fluid therapy some at the discretion of the attending physician. Profound hyperglycaemia developed in 26 and marked hyponatremia in 14 (54%). Whereas blood glucose and serum sodium remained within normal range in the 6 untreated collapsed runners.

The conclusions drawn from this study were as follows: it was concluded that the majority of collapsed runners are not sufficiently dehydrated to warrant IV fluid therapy. Thus such treatment should be reserved for collapsed runners who have clear biochemical other evidence of dehydration Our results also argue against dehydration as the sole cause of exercise-associated collapse. Therefore other pathophysiological explanations for collapse need to be actively considered.

Our further conclusions are as follows:

When hyponatremia is present but does not cause cerebral or other symptoms, it may be an associated feature rather than the cause of collapse. This conclusion is strengthened by our findings that clinical improvement occurred despite the development of hyponatremia in 54% of the runners who received IV therapy. When initial determinations were made, 9% of collapsed runners had hyponatremia. This is similar to the incidence found previously (I do not have the reference to this unfortunately). A high incidence of hyponatremia was found in non collapsed runners. Whereas runners with symptomatic hyponatremia clearly have fluid overload, the fluid status of those with asymptomatic hyponatremia prior to IV therapy remains uncertain.

Important fluid shifts occur during recovery further reducing serum sodium concentrations. The evidence is that plasma volume increased during recovery regardless of whether or not collapsed runners received IV fluid therapy.

IV therapy exaggerates the normal increase in plasma volume that occurs in collapsed runners and leads to a high incidence of hyponatremia and hyperglycaemia. However, the patients in our study who had hyponatremia improved symptomatically.

Physicians experienced in treating collapsed runners typically prescribe IV fluid for runners whom they consider to be dehydrated but for whom no biochemical evidence of dehydration can be found.

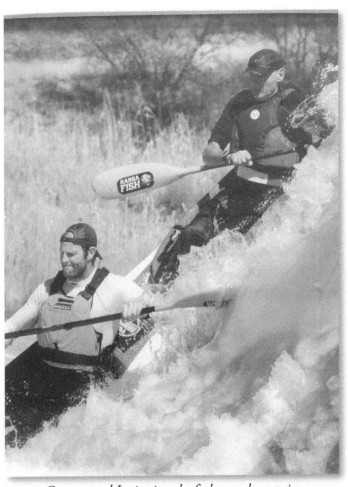

Graeme and I winning the father and son prize
on the FISH RIVER MARATHON-2013
(we won it in1988 for the first time).

A QUAGMIRE IF EVER THERE WAS ONE!

Here I was, literally at the epicentre of the biggest controversy in fluid management to date, where our modus operandi thus far suddenly was in dispute. I had been advocating IV fluid based on well accepted clinical norms of assessment of dehydration and it's management, when the unthinkable reared its ugly head — maybe we had been wrong all along with our fluid management, being far too liberal with dishing out fluids.

One thing I was certain of going forward, and that was assessment of collapsed runners in future was not ever going to be based on actual measurement of blood chemistry, but rather on clinical judgement and hopefully on the judgement of a 'trained eye'. The resources for laboratory investigations at races was not practical. I'm not here referring to elite events such as the Olympics etc where it is mandatory to institute the highest surveillance regarding doping and other indiscretions. Practically speaking most clinicians will have to be satisfied by taking a history and physical examination of the patient in deciding whether to treat dehydration with fluids or not.

Trying to make sense of the differences in Noakes's study compared to what we had been doing successfully for 16 years up to that point, certain differences were immediately discernible. We had started our treatment regime long before it was decided to crank up the amount of fluid we would be ingesting during races to 1 litre per hour. This was only a relatively recent decision and not accepted by everyone. We were using a balanced salt solution in the form of 'Plasmalyte B,' which has the following composition:

magnesium chloride-0.3G/1000ml
potassium chloride 0.3G/1000ml
sodium bicarbonate 2.3G/1000ml
sodium chloride 6G/1000ml

The idea behind using Plasmalyte-B was that it was a balanced salt solution void of glucose which I felt was not needed and would only complicate the clinical picture.

As with most medicines, there a host of side effects that can be attributed to it and Plamalyte-B was no exception, with the ever present diarrhoea and vomiting being listed as possible side effects not to mention muscle cramping, a more tricky discernment to be made when treating collapsed runners. Knowing full well that muscle cramps was listed as a possible side effect, I persisted using it as the muscle cramps that inevitably followed resuscitation, always occurred after the second litre and then magically disappeared as the patient started feeling much better. I attributed this to a return of intra cellular fluid volume which is the area of concern in dehydration. Briefly put, the average 70 kg male has 55 lites of fluid on board, with 5litres in circulation, 15 litres interstitially between the cells and 35 litres intracellularly. It is the fluid in the cells which is first lost as fluid seeps out of the cell into the interstitial fluid which then is used to maintain the circulation which as I said has 5 litres. The circulating 5 litres is vital to maintain supplying the vital organs with oxygen and nutrition and when this becomes inadequate then all sorts of different manifestations of dehydration can occur ranging from mild to severe as discussed earlier.

Tim Noakes was and still is, I am led to understand, adamant that hyponatremia alone is responsible for the collapse of long distance runners and that dehydration per se is not the cause. In my humble opinion, I do not accept this hypothesis. This is based on 17 years of treating collapsed runners in the Two Oceans marathon, using purely clinical signs gained from years of anaesthetic experience when it is crucial and imperative to be able to recognise dehydration accurately. An average of 200 patients per race were treated with IV fluid over the 17 year period, which is 3,400 runners, none of whom experienced adverse effects due to their treatment.

In all the years of administering IV fluid to runners, I only on one occasion caused a serious complication.

One Saturday afternoon I took my son to the beach to do some surfing and on the way home we stopped to watch the finish of a 16 km race taking place in Constantia, the course being a rather testing one with several steep hills. We were standing on the side of the road watching the tail Enders coming in, when I noticed a runners being aided by two other runners. His legs were dragging behind him and the patient looked moribund. I offered to help him after explaining who I was, and we bundled him into a car and took him off to Victoria hospital, a mere kilometre away.

In the A and E, I lay him down and assessed his condition. He was moderately dehydrated but more concerning was his state of alertness. He was semi comatose. I gave him a rapid one litre infusion of Ringers lactate, the only fluid available at the time. Within a few minutes the patient started coughing and soon was coughing up pink frothy sputum. I had pushed the patient into pulmonary oedema, needing immediate oxygen therapy plus furosemide and CPAP (continuous positive airway pressure), until he improved over the next hour. A frightening experience for sure!

Back to the Two Oceans.

An incident occurred in the tent during one of the last races I was involved in, after the findings of Noakes, namely hyponatremia being the main cause for collapse in these runners.

Tim again wanted to conduct more work on runners which of course I agreed to. About midday, a runner was brought in to the tent unconscious and Tim was keen to take over management of the patient. His team got to work on the patient by lifting the patient's legs while we carried on triaging the onslaught of dehydrated runners now coming in to the tent in large numbers. The day became progressively warmer. At some stage I looked over to Tim's corner where the patient still hadn't recovered consciousness fully neither had he been given any IV fluid. I was concerned and asked Tim how long he was going to wait till deciding on fluid. He was not concerned and continued with leg elevation.

Several hours passed and close to half past three in the afternoon, we had cleared the tent of all the runners except for the patient that Tim was busy with. I felt uncomfortable about this situation but was not prepared to get involved with the patient's management at this late stage and left to go home.

Around seven in the evening I was phoned by Chet Sainsbury, the organiser of the race, who was deeply concerned by a phone call he had received from the club chairman of a running club on the East Rand. Apparently he saw on the TV a runner from his club, being taken off to hospital from the Two Oceans grounds, and was worried about his wellbeing which was fully understandable. Chet needed to know what was happening.

I made it perfectly clear to Chet that I was not responsible for the patient's management and that he was under Tim and his team's care. I needed there to be no doubt about this. I had never been queried or challenged by a disgruntled runner, unhappy about their treatment received from me or my staff at the tent. I immediately started phoning the nearby hospitals without any luck. No patient by the name given to me by Chet was admitted to any other hospitals. I told Chet I would contact every hospital in the Cape Peninsula early on Sunday. I phoned all of them without any success.

I decided the best thing to do was to head off to GSH, my teaching hospital and the most likely place a seriously ill patient should be taken. Of course he might be lying in a government morgue Lord forbid, Off to GSH I drove. I asked at casualty if a Mr X was admitted but drew a blank once more.

It struck me that he might have been admitted as an unknown patient in which case he would be known as 'Unknown Saturday' No. 1 or 2 or whatever. Eventually I found the patient in the renal ICU as Unknown Saturday No 6. He had been admitted to the renal unit where he was being monitored. He has received a central venous catheter and needed *ELEVEN LITRES OF FLUID* ! So much for fluid overload.

The above incident upset me deeply. I shudder to think what damage could have ensued. Acute tubular necrosis comes to mind, something I personally was scared of developing way back in 1975 at the Comrades marathon, which is why I opted to give myself at least two litres of fluid at the time.

I regret never having taken the matter up with Tim, an absolute failure on my behalf I am sorry to say. However it made a deep impression on me. I will never accept the fact that all runners who collapse are over hydrated. Some surely are, but the vast majority I have no doubt are depleted. The science needs a lot more elucidation before one definitive cause can take the blame. I don't want to labour the point, we can agree to disagree and leave it there. I will end this discussion by saying that whatever conclusion we come to, it must be in the patient's interests and wellbeing and not for our own gratification that we do what we do as physicians and nurses.

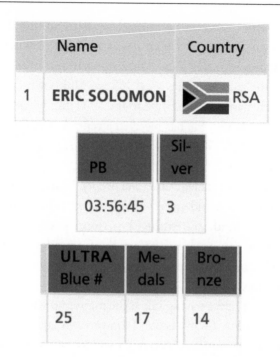

	Name	Country
1	**ERIC SOLOMON**	RSA

PB	Sil-ver
03:56:45	3

ULTRA Blue #	Me-dals	Bro-nze
25	17	14

My Two Oceans running record over 17 years

I would go onto eventually complete 102 marathons, including the seven Comrades and 17 Two Oceans marathons. These I would run mostly in South Africa, the rest being run in Australia(one in 1979 in Sydney), Israel (5 in Jerusalem and 5 in Tiberius-1994-1999) and one in Dublin, Ireland.

Runners high-what is it all about?

The concept of 'runners high' I first heard about in the late 1970s. Non runners were quick to point out that the reason we ran was to experience the 'runners high'. To tell the truth I had no idea what a runner's high would feel like if ever I experienced it yet many runners gloated over the fact that they often experienced it. I soon realised that they were like the blokes who bragged about how often they had sex, were most probably not getting it as often as they claimed they were.

To say that running was always pleasurable was not true. Clearly the experiences of pushing one's body to the extreme in long races were most unpleasant. There were days as well where the run started off poorly and got worse the further one ran. A lot had to do with ones mental state at the time, whether we were tired or hungry or suffering from the after effects of over training which I recognised in my own training program. I was reluctant to give it a break when not feeling up to running and always looked for reasons to continue training, fearing the loss of fitness with even the shortest break, which in retrospect was pathological. I have no doubt that I was fanatical in my approach to running. I suppose it could be labelled an addiction and I'm not going to deny it. However I am not an addictive type of person as I never ever let a craving run away with me, well hardly ever. The truth be told, I love chocolate and behave myself for long periods at a time. But during the hectic training years, I would suddenly go on a binging spree, gorging my self to the point of bursting. Regarding chocolate I could never eat one small square like normal people are meant to do.

Unfortunately chocolate is the one vice that if I break down which is seldom, then there is no stopping my gluttony. It's all or none for me I'm afraid! Fortunately on the other hand, this craving has never applied to other substances such as alcohol, something I enjoy but don't mind if I don't have a drink for months. I have never been tempted to try any form of drug, this has always been a no-no and has never had any appeal what so ever, besides being an anaesthetist with easy access to the most powerful agents on earth, getting involved in substance abuse is a potential death sentence. I love life too much to dabble in such a dangerous game.

Getting back to the runners high, in the mid eighties when I had reached a reasonable level in running, I was able to take on more demanding runs, not that the races such as Comrades and Two Oceans weren't demanding. They were just not conducive to experiencing a runners high. To experience it I thought that many factors were needed to come together to experience the high.

On a late summers evening in Cape Town I decided to go for a run from Constantia neck to the top of the 12 apostles, the mountain range overlooking the Atlantic seaboard adjacent and contiguous with the famous Table Mountain. I enjoyed the solitude of running alone and besides I was feeling pretty good. I set off up the jeep track which would take me to the two dams on the back side of Table Mountain and then headed west till I reached the edge of the escarpment. The sight that greeted me was exquisite - I could see for miles out to sea from this elevation which was about 1000 metres above sea level. The sight was memorable. From there it is possible to see the curvature of the earth and it allowed me to suddenly realise the grandeur of mother nature in full. If ever I experienced a spiritual moment, this was it. At times like this it is difficult not to imagine a greater power controlling this magnificent world, or as Albert Einstein called it "A Cosmic Religious Feeling". I felt elated.

I needed to make tracks as the light was beginning to diminish and I wasn't planning to be caught up on the mountain in the dark, a most undesirable situation to find oneself in. Living in Cape Town I was aware of the statistics of people who succumbed on the mountain, at least 7 lives lost per year on Table Mountain alone. I started running with the sun at my back, my striding body chasing my elongated shadow as I made my way down. I was running effortlessly and was hardly breathing. My mind drifted into a dreamworld where I felt as if I was on a cloud.

Suddenly I was standing near my car parked near the restaurant at Constantia neck where I had started my 20 km run. I have no recall of coming down the mountain whatsoever. I had just experienced a runners high. Endorphins had flooded my body and mind allowing me to join the club of those runners lucky enough to experience the so-called 'runners high'. I had arrived finally!

RUNNING INJURIES I HAVE EXPERIENCED

I have alluded to some of the cardiac events previously, but I feel it is pertinent to repeat them here collectively in order to make clear my cardiac history, describing events that plagued me for many years. This will form the background to me experiencing an episode in 2020 which I clearly could have done without.

Before I get into the details, I want to go through the many so-called mechanical injuries I experienced throughout my running career, which are many, some more sinister than others.

Starting with the lower limb, I'd say tendinitis was the most common over use problem I encountered. The most incapacitating was surely plantar fasciitis, which made getting out of bed in the mornings a nightmare. Running with this condition was not an option and it took time to heal which to any runner is frustrating. I was never keen on taking anti inflammatories (NSAIDS) if I could help it, but rather stuck to the tried and tested treatment of icing, elevation and resting. I never resorted to injecting local anaesthetics (LA) and only used NSAID's when absolutely necessary. I have a healthy respect for these powerful agents and have seen the tragic results of misuse of these agents. A case I recall was of a twenty something year old patient succumbing from total body failure after a dentist injudiciously prescribed a month's supply of NSAIDS for continued use after dental work.

Aches and pain in the feet was not considered to be pathological and was thought to be ware and tare par for the course in runners. In hind sight it was most likely to do with uric acid deposition. I say this because it is becoming abundantly clear that gout per se is more common than previously thought. Instead of the classic picture of a wealthy, opulently obese male who imbibes plenty of alcohol, we are now seeing lesser forms of the condition even in elite well trained athletes who display hardly elevated uric acid levels. Apparently, uric acid has the tendency to deposit in joints exposed to injury. The big toe is not the only joint affected.

Achilles tendonitis was one that I experienced several times but learned to back off quickly and rest till it disappeared. Ignoring the signs of pain followed by crepitus, the feeling of 'bubbles' under the skin was a sure sign that rupture of the tendon was imminent if one persisted with training. A friend of mine suffered this rupture and I was called upon to anaesthetise him for a surgical repair.

Blisters were a continual problem throughout my running career, till I met Tim Noakes who introduced me to 'knee highs', which to the uninitiated are ladies nylon stockings. These were amongst the greatest discoveries I made in my life time. I never saw another blister after using these nylons. I had to endure a lot of mockery from runners and friend regarding my use of these, from cross dressing to you name it. However, it was water off a duck's back, I couldn't have cared less, it worked a charm!

Blisters elsewhere were also problematic and not helped by the stocking. I refer to 'Joggers nipples', a particularly uncomfortable injury from one's T-shirt or vest rubbing on the nipples. This required application of a pre run plaster or a large dollop of vaseline on each nipple or cutting away a portion of the vest to avoid contact.

Chaffing of armpits and between the thighs usually became less of a problem the more my running improved, by body fat content decreased and as a result caused less localised friction.

A running injury I experienced during the late 70's when upping the intensity of my training was a disruption of tendon fibres at the insertion of the adductor muscles on the lower border of the lower pelvic bone, the muscles then inserting distally, to the lower femur around the knee. This condition is commonly referred to as Adductor tendonopathy and took a very long time to disappear. It was an injury I refused to stop running for as it reared its ugly head right in the middle of training for the two ultra marathons which come up in April and May. It never quit left me during this phase of running but finally disappeared as most injuries tend to do.

I will not attempt a full classification of running injuries, as the text books are plentiful and describe to conditions well. I will mention the conditions that were worrisome, and here the iliotibial band (ITB) injury comes to mind. I suffered this at least five times in my career and mainly around the time I was doing serious mileage in the early and mid 80's.

My first experience of ITB was at the end of a 'down' Comrades. I had run what I considered my most comfortable Comrades, feeling good for a large portion of the race miraculously for some unknown reason, but that's how it goes with running. Some things are simply inexplicable. The race was run at a 5minute/km pace, giving me a 7hrs 15minute time and a silver medal to boot. Crossing the line was as usual a good feeling, but on walking off to shower, I felt a severe pain in my left knee, causing me to walk with gait well known to suffered of ITB, namely swinging or rotating one's leg in a circular movement to avoid pain, something I'd seen in plenty of runners but never experienced myself. The pain was no joke. Here NSAIDs were defiantly called for.

The injury is an over use injury where the tensor fascia lata muscle down the lateral side of the thigh, moves repetitively over the femoral lateral epicondyle, causing frictional rubbing particularly on downhill running (as was the case with me). There are several theories on the causation, but suffice to say overuse is paramount amongst these causes. It is an injury which defiantly has the propensity to stop you in your tracks.

Some runners who were unable to accept the inevitable, opted to ignore common sense and sought a surgical answer to the problem. A small cut through the IT band under LA would snip away the few fibres of the band over the epicondyle, in so doing removing the pressure on the condyle. This was a bad idea as was surgically trying to correct a dehiscence of the symphysis pubis, which tragically ended the running career of Errol all those years ago.

A not too common running injury

Heading out for a short 10 km run after work one evening in summer, I was on the home stretch after completing a few circuits in the nearby forest. Nearing home I started experiencing an unpleasant feeling in my bladder. I had emptied it prior to running but didn't drink before the run. On reaching home I went to the toilet and to my absolute horror, my urine was bloody and urinating decidedly unpleasant.

After reading up on the causes of haematuria in runners, I became aware for the first time of this condition labelled 'joggers bladder' which at that stage, I'd not heard of. It is thought that the detrusor muscle of the roof of the bladder hammers down on the neck of the bladder resulting in trauma to the tissues with bleeding as a result. This is more likely to occur when the bladder is empty.

> *LESSON 6: Always have something*
> *to drink before going for a run!*

For peace of mind, I payed the price by having to endure a cystoscopy which proved negative. It was the first and hopefully the last time I would experience joggers bladder.

Running injuries I nearly sustained. What the hell am I talking about? Well, actually I am referring to the birds and seagulls in particular.

On several occasions whilst running on the beach front in Sea Point, the western seaboard of Cape Town, I was attacked by several seagulls, intent to do harm as they dive bombed towards my head. I knew two runners who were actually injured (not seriously though) when attacked by these bird.

The other injury I luckily avoided, but came close to, was *frostbite of the penis.* I kid you not. I moved to Sweden in 2010 after having worked in South Africa for 25 years, I then worked for the next 8 years in the Middle East, followed by 10 years in Ireland, and finally moving to Sweden where my wife was born, where I experienced running in extremely low temperatures for the first time.

Living in the countryside during a fine winter is exhilarating to say the least, with thick powder snow on the ground, bright sunshine in a clear blue sky reflecting off the white snow can only be described as spectacular. Sun glasses are a definite must, it goes without saying.

On a particular day the mercury dropped to minus 26 degrees Celsius, the record low for me at the time. I wasn't really sure how to dress for the occasion. I put on the three recommended layers but didn't wear double lining running longs.

I set out to run a 10 km run in the forest which was memorable, a winter wonder land if ever I saw one. On returning home, I undressed and noticed that I couldn't feel my 'willie' at all, a very strange sensation altogether. It was as if it was anaesthetised. Suddenly the thought struck me it could be frost bite! Surly not, but then I was clueless as to how it felt. Fortunately feeling returned after a while and going forward I decided to pad my nether regions with cotton wool prior to embarking on any runs at low temperatures.

Coincidental injuries

I will end this off by mentioning an incident which could have ended badly. I was running down a mountain path some twenty years ago when I came upon several boxes of bees placed there by a beekeeper. I was no nearer than 20 meters away from the hives when on mass, a swarm of bees suddenly attacking me unprovoked. I fled from the area tearing my running vest off my body and swinging wildly trying to disperse the bees, only partially successfully. I ended up with 25 bee stings on my chest, head and neck, a most painful and unpleasant experience indeed. Fortunately I am not allergic to bee stings

Problems related to the Cardiovascular System

I have alluded to some of the cardiac events previously, but I feel it is pertinent to repeat them here collectively in order to make clear my cardiac history, in describing events that plagued me for many years, resulting in me experiencing an episode I clearly could have done without.

Our training in Anaesthesia in South Africa and particularly in CapeTown at the famous Groote Schuur Hospital was thorough. We were fortunate to have spend a fair amount of time doing cardiac anaesthesia at a time when South Africa was up there with the best in the world, at least Groote Schuur was thanks to professor Christaan Barnard who put cardiac surgery on the world map. We were expected to have a good understanding of ECG's as we dealt with situations not normally seen in non cardiac procedures. Cases out of the ordinary included double heart transplants, where the recipient retained his own heart whilst receiving a donor heart from another patient. Initially the two hearts were paced to work together, but later on they were left to beat unpaced. Earlier on in the book I referred to a 'cardiectomy' where a patient with HOCM had his transplanted heart removed due to rejection, once more having to be reliant on his own heart which, it was hoped, had recovered amply to maintain an adequate circulation.

In truth, during my 45years of administering anaesthesia to 86,000 patients, I saw many arrhythmias in patients during that time, very few of which were sinister thank goodness. The majority of arrhythmias were sinus arrhythmias, with bradycardia denoting a vagal response or drug related causes or more serious, severe anoxia especially in children. Sinus tachycardia usually called for deepening anaesthesia or checking to see that a drug was not inadvertently administered. Atrial arrhythmias were more common with AF - atrial fibrillation often being difficult to manage depending on its duration. Then there were the junctional and re-entry tachycardias that were not too common, but needed active intervention all the same. Escape rhythms, which were a safety response to failure of the SA node to fire. Ectopic beats on the other hand, appeared earlier than expected. These are also known as extrasystoles or premature beats. These were ubiquitous, often being benign in nature.

When one of these beats originated in the ventricles, we would sit up and take note, as some were in need of management, depending if they were single or not, unifocal or multifocal and depending on their frequency.

Very infrequently, I had patients who developed

VT - ventricular tachycardia, which implied a potentially sinister arrhythmia which could easily go on to VF, ventricular fibrillation, the anaesthetists ultimate nightmare, up there with CVCO (can't ventilate/can't oxygenate)! Fortunately every case of VT that my patients developed, was successfully treated with cardioversion. The only case that tragically ended in ventricular fibrillation was a case I anaesthetised in the late 1980s where the patient's core temperature fell below 32 degrees centigrade despite my every effort to raise the temperature. Unfortunately the cold heart is usually unresponsive to drugs and we lost the patient.

This brings me to my own personal experience with arrhythmias, which had its origins years ago and continued throughout my adult life to the present time.

I took up running at the age of 28 when I was a general practitioner to lose some weight. It worked well and I lost weight to the extent that my weight returned to what I weighed at high school.

My resting pulse rate also started slowing down and I managed to reach a low of 46/min, a sort of reward for all the hard work. But there it stayed and stand on my head, I couldn't go below 46 beats a minute, until I left Benoni on the East Rand, not too far from Johannesburg and headed down to Cape Town to specialise in anaesthesia in 1975. With all the running I did in the Cape, up and down Table Mountain (1000 meters), my resting pulse soon drifted into the mdid 30's, and I was particularly proud of the fact that on one occasion it hit a low of 32 beats/min.

My new low resting pulse rate seemed innocuous enough, but I did notice the onset of extra beats, mainly

VEB's(ventricular extrasystoles) and mainly unifocal. None of this stopped me from running and I felt well for years despite the persistent reminders.

On one occasion in the mid 80's, I took part in a 24 hour relay race which was quite exhausting. The next day I felt so-called 'cannon waves' in my neck, a rather uncomfortable feeling indeed. After the days work in theatre, I did my own ECG and discovered to my horror that it was definitely abnormal, not exactly clear as to what was potting. I went off to see our professor of cardiology, prof Wally Beck, who ordered another ECG and echo cardiogram. It appears he was thinking I might have HOCM, hypertrophic obstructive cardiomyopathy. My heart sank, I thought my life was over, let alone my running career. Merrily it turned out to be less sinister. I had a well trained heart as seen in Bushmen in the Kalahari and African miners working 4 km deep in the South African gold mines, according to the professor.

I learned to live with these VEB's and despite even experiencing them in races, I never had any adverse effects such as dizziness, dyspnea, or chest pain.

During 2005 whilst working in Ireland, Eva my wife and I decided to partake in a 10 km fundraiser race in County Clare. The race was more a fun run, so I didn't see the need to warm up despite the race starting off up a steep hill. One hundred meters from the start I needed to stop as I felt I was out of breath. My wife asked what the matter was and I replied that it felt my pulse had not increased as it should have with the sudden increase of activity. I started off again slowly and within one km I was back to my old self and I sped off like in the good old days. After this on several occasions, I noticed that it would be a while after starting to run, that my heart rate would speed up and only then that I could run as fast as I like.

Fast forward to 2014 and a similar episode occurred while on holiday in Cape Town. Eva persuaded me to see a cardiologist, so I visited an old friend Joe Tyrrell, who was a running friend from the past as well as a fine cardiologist. Joe put me on a 24 hour cardiac holter, followed up by an ultrasound of the heart, and CT angiogram to rule out a silent myocardial infarct, all of which proved negative. I was relieved to know my heart's structure was normal and my coronary vessels clear with a calcium score of 8.4, fortunately extremely low for a 71 year old. The consensus when discussing my problem with two electrophysiologists was that I most probably suffered from *idiopathic ventricular ectopy,* something I was not too aware of at this stage (but later would become extremely aware of and its significance). They suggested taking a beta blocker, Metoprolol, but I was extremely reluctant to do so as I already had a resting pulse rate of 35/min.

After this I returned to Sweden where I had finally decided to hang up my running shoes, well not actually hang them up, but rather run no more than 4-5 km at a time. I started riding a trail bike which I found was kinder on the knees and hips, which were fine still. Mind you, I was getting strange flitting aches and pains in my feet which appeared related to running. I was loving the bike as I got plenty exercise and didn't feel wrecked after a two hour ride. Besides, here I was getting good cardiovascular exercise and being able to keep a strict watch on my heart rate with my GPS watch which was a pulse meter as well.

One day at the end of April 2020 I rode a testing 30 kms

on my mountain bike and was feeling good afterwards with nothing hurting which is always a bonus. The next day, Eva and I, with our Golden Retriever dog Dougal, set out for a routine 6 km round walk which included a steep hill in the nearby forest. Clearly I hadn't fully recovered from the ride the day before despite no stiffness. My legs felt it somewhat, the sort of feeling I learned to recognised when the glucose stores in the muscles and liver had not sufficiently recovered. Added to this I missed out on lunch which I substituted with a large mug of very strong Swedish, full roast coffee sans sugar.

We were on the home stretch, one kilometre from home when Eva and I both blurted out simultaneously that we felt somewhat hypoglycaemic. Dougal was unusually perky at this stage and I had him on the lead and needed to therefore trot behind him. It was at this stage that I suddenly had to stop. I felt that I had run out of steam. I lowered my head and put my hands on my knees. I felt my radial pulse which was extremely thready. I was unable to count it as it was so rapid. I had no other symptoms such as chest pain or shortness of breath or dizziness. I hitched a ride home where I lay down and took my pulse and blood pressure. Pulse was 215/min and the BP 105 /65 mmHg. I immediately tried carotid artery massage and the Valsalva manoeuvre, both to no avail.

I was worried. Eva suggested calling the ambulance but I was hesitant. I said let us give it 10 minutes more and see if it stops. It didn't. When the ambulance arrived the crew did an ECG. I asked to look at it. I immediately looked at the widened QRS complexes and looked for P-waves which weren't visible. Could this be a VT (ventricular tachycardia)?

I hoped that it could be a wide QRS complex AVNRT (AV nodal re-entry tachycardia) with a partial heart block pattern, being far less ominous than VT.

Once in the hospital the sustained tachycardia settled with IV Adenosine, indicating that the arrhythmia was most likely an AVNRT. Three months went by and I assumed it was a one-off episode, but I was bitterly disappointed when it occurred four more times within a three week period. I was becoming paranoid. The treatment for each of the episodes was different. Adenosine ceased to be effective. They reverted to cardioversion which worked twice, once it reverted by itself spontaneously and the last episode only reverted back to sinus rhythm with the agent Amioderone (Corderone), usually reserved for ventricular arrhythmias.

The second last episode of VT prior to undergoing ablation, occurred when we were hiking though a beautiful nature reserve. We had just completed 8 km of hill walking, when all of a sudden the arrhythmia started, VT in all its glory. We still had to negotiated a steep hill of 1.5 km, and it was getting dark. My options were limited so I managed to climb the hill without dizziness, chest pain or shortness of breath with a pulse rate of over 200/minute at the age of 76years. I must have reasonably good effort tolerance and cardiac reserve. The VT didn't kill me thank goodness! Fortunately the VT reverted back to a sinus rhythm without intervention.

It was decided that I needed to go to Örebro for a possible ablation of the heart. I could hardly believe that my heart, which I had nurtured all these years was suddenly developing sustained tachycardia and my body was about to be invaded to resolve the issue. I could hardly take this all in.

The day dawned in early November 2020, and I arrived in the radiology suit where the ablation was to take place. I was briefed in characteristic Swedish style, namely quietly, orderly and unambiguously to what I could expect. Without further ado, I was wheeled in and they proceeded to work on me. A young (by my standards) doctor approached my right groin with local anaesthesia and with only feeling a bit of pressure, he inserted the various catheters through the femoral vein into the right atrium.

No sooner had this been done when I instantly recognised the unpleasantness of rapid pulsations in the neck and awareness of my abdominal aorta tapping against the paper towels covering me fro tip to toe. Out the corner of my eye I could just see the screen which clearly showed a tracing of what I had learn to recognise as the broad QRS complexes of VT.

There was a palpable urgency as they tried to slow it down, apparently unsuccessfully with drugs. They had as yet not even started with the mapping of the heart waiting to first arrest the tachycardia. They decided to electro-cardiovert me. A young female anaesthetist approached me from behind and placed an Ambu-bag mask on my face. I tried to breath but the system she was using had an expiratory valved closed instead of fully opened. The pressure was rapidly building up in my airway and lungs and the anaesthetist was completely oblivious of this situation. All the while no response from the anaesthetist as I thrashed my head from side to side gasping for air. I showed my displeasure at her lack of sensitivity but soon lost consciousness as the anaesthetic took effect. I was shocked seven times apparently, each time the heart starting off in sinus rhythm but rapidly reverting back into VT. (As an anecdote, I have to say that the poor judgement displayed by the anaesthetist in not recognising my plight was the antithesis of the rest of my treatment which was magnificent to say the least.)

During one of my lucid periods they inserted a temporary pacemaker into the heart via the neck veins on the right side as well as an arterial line in the right radial artery in order to do an angiogram of the coronaries which were thankfully still patent as they were five years ago with the CT angiogram I had in Cape Town all to rule out coronary artery disease as a cause for sustained VT.

I was sent back to the thoracic ICU where it was later explained to me what had transpired. Apparently my pulse had gone down to 25beats/min-certainly my all time record.

After the majority of my veins in both arms were utilised for the various procedures, I looked at my arms which had never been subjected to this sort of treatment before.

The next day I was wheeled into the suit once more and this time things proceeded in a far more relaxed fashion. The mapping of the Right Atrium showed no abnormality and conduction down the AV node was normal. The problem clearly was not in the atria, neither did I have an AVNRT. They advanced the mapping process into the right ventricle and saw immediately that the source of the ectopy lay in the lateral wall of the right ventricle, close to a cusp of the tricuspid valve. This is called Idiopathic ventricular ectopy for lack of a more specific term. The site was ablated and tested afterwards by giving me atropine and isoprenaline to try and elicit a tachycardia response, which fortunately did not occur.

They had successfully ablated the cause of my VT They were extremely happy with their management but not as happy as I was. My only remaining concern was what could have caused this abnormal site of excitation? Later, after having read about several other cases in well trained hearts, it has become clear that 'stretch' injuries from over distention of the myocardium with the sort of extreme running up steep gradients, which I relished, was in all probability responsible in part for the damage.

It was decided, because my pulse rate was tending to be in the lower 30's, that my SA node was getting 'lazy' and sooner or later I would need a pacemaker. So without further ado, they inserted Boston Scientific pacemaker (AAI with DDD backup), suitable for an active person which I still hoped to be after this ordeal.

What I learned from this entire episode was that it is possible to live an active life for many years with arrhythmias as long as they were not sinister. I was under the impression that VT was always dangerous. However VT without structural heart disease (5%of cases) is not the same as VT with structural disease(95%). Their outcomes differ vastly which doesn't mean to say one should ever take VT lightly.

It took me 45 years of varied anaesthetic practice to finally get to experience VT first hand. It is a valuable lesson when caring for patients with arrhythmias. It is information I feel is necessary to share with colleagues who might not have come across this in their practices. The whole experience has led me to become interested in electrophysiology, which has changed dramatically since I studied physiology for the primary examination of the fellowship in anaesthesia, way back in in1974. Fortunately I retained a keen interest in medicine and anaesthesia all these years and tried to remain current at all times.

It is becoming blatantly clear that years of heavy training of the sort I partook in, can possibly have deleterious effects not only on joints, but on the heart as well. I chose to do a lot of training on hills, the steeper the better. This in turn was the reason for my pulse rate fluctuating in the lower 30's for most of the time. What I was oblivious of was the damage being inflicted on my myocardium in the form of excessive myocardial stretching, possibly causing micro tears and bleeding, leading to healing by fibrosis. One of these scarred areas might just have been the exact cause of my monomorphic *idiopathic ventricular ectopy.*

I subsequently read a book entitled "The Haywired Heart"-How too much exercise can kill you, and what you can do to protect your heart, by Chris Case, John Mandrola and Lennard Zinn, where elite cyclists and electro cardiologists collate the findings in several top class athletes who suffered similar fates. This emerging information should be taken seriously. More it seems, might not be better than less when it come to exercise.

The way I rationalise my situation is as follows. Having exercised heavily for many years, I like to think that by doing the sort of 'cardio-protective ' exercise of hill running, and so reducing my resting pulse drastically, I therefore protected my heart from the usual pathologies so prevalent in western society today. Unfortunately I fell victim to the complications of excessive exercise which happens in trained athletes, namely scarring. I was fortunate to avoid the most serious of complications seen in patients with VT, namely VF, which apparently seldom happens to the small percentage of exercisers due to their preserved myocardium.

As can be seen, the situation can be summed up as follows-'Dammed if you do, and dammed if you don't!'

Time will tell…

PART TWO

HOW MY DIET CHANGED THROUGHOUT MY RUNNING CAREER

At the outset I want to make it perfectly clear that I am not trained as a nutritionist and never claimed to be an expert on nutrition or diet. What I describe here is not in any way meant to decry research done by so-called experts. All I have done is to look objectively at all past and current thoughts on nutrition, draw what seems reasonable and rational from them, and apply it to my own way of eating.

As a child growing up in South Africa during the Apartheid years, I was fortunate to have grown up in a caring family of modest income, able to feed us sufficiently. I dare say that what we ate was similar to the lifestyle of our grandparents who originally came from Lithuania. They did not have the luxury of choice that we have today. Meat and fatty meat at that, was a staple in their diet, plus white bread home baked, was eaten with every meal for sure. Dairy played an important part and provided a good source of protein.

From a very early age I displayed a dislike for fat and dairy products. This is one of my definite childhood memories. It has never changed. It is strange indeed that I alone in the family adopted this aversion to fats and dairy. Nobody influenced me in my choice, I knew nobody else with my ideas. I developed an intolerance to milk which I rarely drank. On a very hot day spent on the beach in Cape Town during the end of year vacation after second year of my medical studies in1964, I downed a pint of milk rapidly as that's all that was available. It didn't take very long to pass right through me. I wasn't at all surprised, and the incident confirmed my aversion to dairy products as being fully rational.

I have to make an admission about some idiosyncrasies I displayed as a teenager. I had a rapacious appetite for eating which put most other peers to shame. My brother, six year my senior, would take bets with his friends in regard to my notorious eating habits. Two examples were ingesting 45 bananas in one sitting and on another occasion eating an entire chocolate cake in one sitting to win a bet for my brother. My parents were unaware of such idiotic behaviour from their youngest. Even today I shudder to think of how ridiculous (and dangerous what's more) that was. Yet I survived to tell the tale.

Fast forward to the early seventies, and I find myself in general practice as a family doctor where we were expected to give advice on most matters pertaining to well being. Our knowledge was limited but there were guideline set out that we followed which seemed rational at the time. The one thing I will say though, is that we were well trained to examine patients fully and take detailed histories which went a long way in making a diagnosis. However ability to curing patients from many conditions was limited. High blood pressure, a very common condition, was poorly treated as there was relatively slow progress in development of newer drugs to manage the condition. Likewise drugs to treat heart disease was also slow. So called ACE inhibitors, to treat blood pressure were yet to be discovered, beta blockers on the other hand appeared in the early seventies and played a large roll. Diabetes, ubiquitous then as now, the nemesis of all practitioners and patients was not an easy condition to manage despite having a good idea of the pathophysiology of the disease. I mention this specifically as I allude to the micro vascular pathology seen specifically in diabetes which is unlike that of most other conditions affecting the vascular system where the pathology lies mainly in the larger vessels. So that was more or less the situation in medicine at the time I started running and of course I needed to reduce weight considerably at the same time.

I mentioned earlier on in the book that patients complaining of tiredness and lethargy would get a lecture from me on the benefits of exercising, not that I was doing anything about the problem myself. Weight loss advice was to inform the patient to do the obvious and that was to eat less, as well as to eat 'healthily' what ever that meant as well as exercise, poorly defined then. I assumed at the time it meant cut down on fatty food and less sweet stuff, nothing too specific at all. If the patient had heart disease or if there was any heart disease in the family, then it was important to reduce animal fats, triglycerides and cholesterol and trans fats in general. After all familial combined hyperlipidaemia was well known, and often led to early demise from heart attacks in families. We even had a chap in our final year class who died a few years after qualifying, who had this condition in the family. To me there was no doubt about this link with lipids and heart disease, but the picture was far from clear then as it is still to this day I'm sad to relate. Why this is so difficult to solve remains a mystery. Millions have been spent on finding the cause of CVD yet the definitive answer remain elusive.

My own metamorphosis regarding weight loss started from the day I decided to start running. The initial weight loss was dramatic within a few weeks, solely due to eating much less and not changing my diet in any other way. A simple decrease in food intake, full stop. I continued to avoid dairy and eggs but continued eating meat, always cutting off the excessive visible fat. Barbecuing in SA is a national preoccupation where sausage (boereworse), steak, lamb chops can be found everywhere on weekends, folk gathered around the grill whilst eating huge amounts of fatty meat, washed down by litres of beer and brandy spirits while discussing the merits of the Springbok rugby team's performance at the last outing (Springboks team is the national rugby team of SA). It was difficult to avoid meat all together at this stage I will confess.

The other foodstuff I need to mention is something called 'Biltong', which is game meat that is salted and hung up to dry, leaving a delightfully flavoured meat preserve, a relic from the past when the Voortrekkers of old had no refrigeration on their long trek from the Cape Colony to the hinterland in wagons to escape the domination of the British who had usurped control in the southern tip of Africa in 1795, heralding the ending of the Dutch East India Company's control in the Cape.

This Biltong delicacy was generally lean meat from a variety of buck notably the Kudu or Impala, but the ubiquitous Springbok biltong was the stuff legends were made of. Springbok biltong is part of the genetic make up of South Africans, which I hazard a guess might have something to do with the endemic prevalence of heart disease in White South Africans.

As a medical student, I recall clearly that if one mentioned myocardial infarction as a possible cause of death in an African patient, you would fail the exam not to mention be laughed at. It simply wasn't seen in Africans until they started eating similar food to the caucasians when their economic situation improved toward the end of the apartheid era. The 'coloured' population(mixed race population) on the other hand suffered the same amount of heart disease if not more than whites. The propensity for developing certain diseases was clearly different in the different racial groups. For example malignant hypertension was prevalent in blacks, more so than whites. But I digress.

So I had no compunction in advising patients to limit fat intake. A few years later after I left general practice to specialise in anaesthetics, looking at studies where groups of different ethnicities were compared, it seemed to follow the same pattern. In the mid seventies while I was studying for my part two of the anaesthetic exam, I came upon an article comparing an Arab cohort to a group of Israelis of Ashkenazi origin. I don't recall any details of the study except the outcome which seem to point to a decidedly higher incidence of Coronary Artery disease in the Jewish cohort compared to the Arab group despite the fact that the Arab group were by far heavier smokers compared to the Ashkenazi group in this study. It was put down possibly to the dietary differences.

A CHANGE IS ABOUT TO TAKE PLACE

In 1977 after completing my exams to become a specialist anaesthetist, I was attending a military camp in the Cape as commanding officer of 20 Field Ambulance Battalion, a citizen force unit in the SADF (SA defence force) designated a non conventional field ambulance by virtue of how we operated.

We were to spend a month in the bush on exercises meant to replicate bush warfare that SA was involved in up in the northern sector of South West Africa, later called Namibia, as well as Angola, the so called Border War, that raged between 1966-1989.

The exercise took place in October/November of 1977, a most memorable year for a variety of reasons one of which was that my youngest daughter was born shortly before the training camp was to begin. The weather during the camp was hot and the Western Cape was experiencing a severe drought which created several logistical problems one of which was that the cooler trucks carrying food stores often broke down leading to destruction of several food stores. In the main keeping meat fresh proved to be the biggest problem.

The army did its best to provide us with prime meat which was not exactly the sort of food that appealed to me. Inspecting the trucks that were breaking down confirmed my aversion to eating meat. I still recall the unsightly appearance of the fatty meat with a distinct green tinge to it. Nothing, I decided, could be less appetising than the sight of less than fresh meat.

It also happened that the BMJ(British Medical Journal)

at the time ran a series of three articles comparing animal protein to that of plant based protein, a timeous study in deed which was to influence my decision hence forth to stop eating meat altogether. 1977 was the year I ceased to eat meat as such and only ate fish, and when necessary, lean chicken as well. I say necessary on purpose because not everyone in my family agreed with my ideas and restricting them all to fish only I felt would be rather unfair.

To my way of thinking the advantages of eating whole grains and plant based protein, compared to animal protein outweighed the more complete protein content of animal sources, as I sincerely believed that saturated fats which necessarily form part of eating animal protein were not in our best interests.

Meanwhile I continued with my low fat/no fat diet all by myself as far as I knew. The carbo-loading regimen so popular at the time would later become unpopular and be replaced by keto diets, intermittent fasting, LCHF and, horror of horrors, the inappropriate use of medicines specifically designed for the treatment of type-2 diabetes, namely Metformin and the GLP-1RA-receptor agonists, namely 'Semaglutide' which blunts the appetite with the idea of regulating glucose usage and control in the body, all to loose weight. Experts warn however that this is not a quick fix replacement for healthy eating and exercise.

MY SECRET WEAPON

As early as the mid 70's, in fact 1975 to be precise, I started to eat peanut butter in ernest. The reason for my reluctance to really launch into the stuff was that stories were bandied around of raised cholesterol and fats in peanut butter, supposedly as dangerous as fats from animal sources. It took a long time to show these concerns to be spurious and totally unfounded. It is true though that most manufacturers of peanut butter tend to add all sorts of ingredients to improve the taste artificially. I caught onto this at an early stage and sought out only the purest peanut butter devoid of the usual culprits, namely palm oil, sea salt and sugar. Palm oil in particular is a bad additive as it is apparently high in saturated fats which if you believe in the deleterious cardiac effects on the CVS (as I do), then it is to be avoided when possible.

I therefore sought out a source containing no additives, and launched my new found diet, with peanut butter at the centre of my daily nutritional intake. I must clarify here that I 'laid it on thick'. My daily intake might scare the average person not used to such quantities.

My standard breakfast from the time I moved to Cape Town in 1975 to the present day has been the same, I've never tired of it once! It consists of two slices of whole wheat bread with as much peanut butter as I can get between the two slices without overflow onto the table cloth. Nothing else on the sandwich is needed-no butter nor margarine nor any other substance, they are superfluous.

In addition to this I must elucidate further: I would generally run early in the mornings, usually before leaving for work. I wouldn't eat breakfast at home as there wasn't time to do so, besides I wasn't hungry till about 10 o'clock in the morning. This was convenient as we normally broke for a tea break between cases which allowed me to launch into my long awaited calorie loaded sandwich, washed down with a strong cup of black coffee. This has remained my modus operandi till this very day with one exception. I have dispensed with the two teaspoons of sugar I had in the coffee in the old days as here in Sweden where I now reside, we don't use sugar in the coffee which took some getting used to but now is my preferred way of drinking the beverage. Swedes by the way, drink the most coffee per capita in the world.

Several things came together when I started this peanut butter regime. By virtue of only eating at 10 or 11 am each day, suddenly I was only eating two meals instead of the traditional three meals I was used to. This meant that my total calorie intake was down despite the huge amount of peanut butter ingested mid morning. What became evident later on was that I was partaking in intermittent fasting, which became fashionable around 2012, in the form of time-restricted fasting, which involves only eating during certain hours of the day. This I had discovered myself when I started my fad but hadn't realised its significance. My idea was to eat essentially when I was hungry. Running as much as I did made me realise two things about my physiology. The more I ran, the less I needed to eat and the less sleep I needed. It didn't take long in the early 80's to realise what this could lead to. My weight just fell off me and I reached an all time low weight of 76 kg, my height being 193 cm. This translated into a BMI (body mass index) of 20,4(20-25 normal range for males). I looked gaunt and was very sensitive to cold, my low body fat surly contributing to this. One glass of cold water and I needed a pull-over or jersey for sure. Not needing to sleep did worry me because I clearly was not getting enough sleep by all normal accounts, yet I never felt tired or exhausted. Anorexia came to mind but I would never admit that I enjoyed it when people said I was looking terrible. Alternatively, if they said I was looking better, it upset me, it meant I wasn't running enough. One's own body image is complex and hard to define or even less compare objectively with others who view us in a different light.

I have always felt that I have insight into such matters. Being a doctor and anaesthetist means that I need to maintain objectivity if possible. I decided that I needed to throttle back just enough to continue running well without tipping over the line. My weight drifted up slowly to 80 kg and has fluctuated between 80-84kg ever since.

I pride myself in having insight into most things, yet I am not immune to the foibles that beset us all at some stage of our lives. It is difficult to know when one is doing something in excess or not. Who is to judge? Can a non runners cast an opinion? The book is yet to be written as to what is a normal amount of running? All this, I'm afraid is subjective and shall remain so.

Slowly we are learning that too much running might not be good for one.

In summary here I can say that the discovery of pure unadulterated peanut butter as a source of protein and 'good' fat was an epiphany. Here was a nutritious food, cheap and plentiful and something that satisfied my hunger adequately, freeing me up to work and train and forget about food during the day, something that can't be said about many diets and fads. Plus eating it this way, I was able to maintain a decent weight around 80-83kg without having to worry about food all the time.

I must add to this that the satiety generally lasted me till supper time where I ate a decent normal meal but resisted second helpings as a rule, a normal supper was fish/chicken, vegetables inclusive of potatoes, usually boiled but not fries as fries are a no-no in my book. I was never fond of any type of sauce or gravy, preferring food on its simplest form.

What about alcohol you might ask?

I used to drink plenty of beer as a medical student in the 60's. I couldn't afford to buy it, so I brewed my own beer. The process was simple and after just over a week we had a yield of 12 dozen beers. I won't go into the details but we produced sufficient quantities to keep ourselves in a permanent stupor on weekends if desired. Clearly this was unsustainable not to mention unhealthy, but we were very popular at parties on weekends needless to say.

All this ceased when I became a doctor, well almost

ceased as during our intern year, we worked extremely hard, and also when free, we partied hard. When my responsibilities increased, it all stopped. By the time I took up running, alcohol intake was limited, and the beer was replaced by red wine, something I enjoy even today. I am happy to say that I have never had a craving for alcohol and can do without it for extended periods.

One day during the 80's in Cape Town, I was sitting in the tea room of a suburban private hospital, during cases. I had asked for my usual pot of peanut butter and two slices of whole-wheat bread. Rita, a nurse in theatre, brought me the plate with the peanut butter. She asked me how I managed to keep my weight down when I ate such an obscene amount of the stuff. I told her that was all I ate till supper time which I had when I got home. I asked her if she ate breakfast, she answered that she did'nt. I suggested that she give it a try, namely a similar sandwich at 10-11:00 in the morning, then no cheating till supper time when she could have her normal supper without a second helping.

Rita became a convert instantly. She lost 12 kg over a few weeks and never felt hungry during that time. It was then that I knew it was something that could have a wide application. It made complete sense, eating something that was healthy, cheap available worldwide and satisfied ones hunger in the main without needing additives.

Peanut butter paste has been used in Africa to feed starving children cheaply. Marasmus and kwashiorkor, two commonly seen disorders in Southern Africa, result from severe nutritional deficiencies. Peanut butter has a big role to play here.

Headlong into the fray

In recent years a major change in our thinking regarding the effect of food on several major illnesses, has caused us to sit up and rethink our strategies regarding management. The two obvious conditions are Diabetes Mellitus and Coronary Artery disease, both responsible for large numbers of patients in need of support worldwide

The problem is long standing and has been around seemingly forever. Both conditions are well described and virtually any medical practitioner worth his/her salt is able to make the diagnosis when confronted. However, what is not clear is what the actual mechanism or causation of either conditions is.

With diabetes we know that there is a shortage of insulin from the pancreas, absolute or relative and the disease is referred to as type1, which is an immune mediated form of the disease, usually appearing in young people but not always. The other is type 2, which is prevalent in all populations usually living in relative affluent societies. This needs clarification as in poor countries it is a disease of the rich, whereas in affluent countries it tends to be a disease of the poor, although not necessarily so.

It is not the place nor my intention to give a lecture on diabetes, but suffice to say environmental factors play a role. Glucose intolerance together with excessive weight gain is certainly important in the aetiology of diabetes. It is thought that poor early nutrition can predispose to diabetes in later life. What is impaired glucose tolerance? It is characterised by a raised blood glucose which usually can be reversed by a combination of diet and exercise.There are several criteria needed to fit the picture but it is estimated that less than 2% of the population fit this picture of unsuspected diabetes. There is no specific clinical picture to describe this but of importance is that early detection is required as it can lead onto diabetes as well as cardiovascular disease. What is Insulin Resistance?

Here the term refers to the cells of the body being resistant to insulin which then leads to blood glucose levels rising and eventually leading to type 2 diabetes. Obesity is an important factor as well. Insulin resistance is also known as impaired insulin sensitivity, cause unknown, and in time will lead to depletion of the beta-cells of the pancreas to produce insulin leading to type 2 diabetes.

The two above terms are important when considering the disease we call diabetes. Factors playing a role are obesity, a family history, lack of exercise and high blood pressure.

In regard to Insulin resistance, factors that play a role are similar to glucose intolerance, namely, obesity, inactivity, family history, and a diet high in carbohydrates. If the truth be told the terms are somewhat confusing, there is no clearcut delineation. The bottom line is that Diabetes is a condition where supply and demand of insulin becomes unbalanced and we as doctors need to find a way to lower the demands by dietary means if possible. What advice can and should we offer patients who find themselves well on the way to developing type 2 diabetes?

How to go about preventing it where possible is going to be the topic for discussion.

THE BIG CONTROVERSIES

As mentioned, diabetes and cardiovascular share many of the same complications. Anything that can lessen the complications of diabetes will do so for CVD as well.

Controlling the amount of carbohydrates in pre as well as established diabetics is obvious, there can be no question. A total abstinence is not likely to succeed as we depend on carbohydrates as a primary source of energy. There are those who say that man was never meant to eat carbohydrates, but I challenge this hypothesis.

For 2.5 million years humans fed themselves by gathering plants and hunting animals. Some 10,000 years ago they began planting seeds, wheat, peas and lentils. According to Harari (*3),"90%of calories that feed humans come from a handful of plants that our ancestors domesticated between 9500 and 3500 BC.-Wheat rice, maize, potatoes, millet and barley". Then,"As soon as this happened they cheerfully abandoned the gruelling, dangerous, and often spartan life of hunter-gatherers settling down to enjoy the pleasant, satiated life of farmers".

This new agricultural revolution provided more readily available food supplies, which doesn't translate necessarily into better food. I'm not going to discuss the pros and cons or merits of the different foods. All I want to suggest is that mankind has been eating grains and carbohydrates for a very long time.

As an example, we humans posses *Amylase,* in the saliva and pancreas, which is an enzyme solely for the digestion of sugars and starch. I can hardly believe that the enzyme is redundant, put there for no obvious reason. Nature doesn't do such things.

Each molecule of glucose yields 36 ATP's whereas lipid(fat) oxidation provides more ATP but at the cost of needing more oxygen to do so. Therefore both fats and carbohydrates are sources of energy, carbohydrates should not be shunned per se. Reducing carbohydrate intake especially in the indolent is a good idea. It is not rocket science that weight gain increases with high intake and minimal exercise. I believe that the refined sugars are the carbohydrates that should be avoided in both the active and the indolent.

Here I am sticking my neck out. There is a growing consensus (which I do not accept) that the way forward in preventing both diabetes and CVD is to adopt the low carbohydrate/high fat diet, where ideally, carbohydrates are avoided and replaced by fats, excluding triglycerides. Saturated fats are acceptable. This the protagonists will tell you is clearly advantageous and is the way forward.

Ancel Keys, the originator of the-'heart and lipid' hypothesis, said in brief that fats were the cause of heart disease (cholesterol in particular). I am not expanding on this as the literature is enormous. The argument challenging this hypothesis is that Cholesterol has nothing to do with CHD(coronary heart disease), but rather it has very much to do with Insulin resistance, which is made worse by eating carbohydrates rather than fats which Keys said was the cause of the heart disease all those years ago. So poor Keys is blamed for setting the ball rolling by falsely claiming that cholesterol causes CHD, and thereby is responsible for the exponential explosion of type 2 diabetes by inference of eating a diet high in carbohydrates.

I have given a short summary in essence of the battle raging at present between the conventional medical opinion, which still lays blame on fats as being at least partially responsible for the rise in CHD, and the other side, namely the pro Ketone dieters, the Banters and the low/no carbohydrate/high fat/protein(LCHF) dieters.

The problem is extremely complicated and far from being resolved. What I will do is give my interpretation, anecdotally of what I think we should do, based solely on my observations throughout my life as a father, a doctor, anaesthetist and runner. After all, if I didn't learn anything along the way, then I truly wasted my time!

CONCLUSIONS BASED ON MY OBSERVATIONS

At the outset, I have to say that there surely is not only one solution that fits everyone. This is self evident. We are all different and react differently to various diets. This was nowhere more obvious to me that in the administration of anaesthesia. We use guidelines when administering agents to patients but one has to be cognisant of possible differences in response to the agents. Older patients usually need less and the robust more but this could prove to be just the opposite as the elderly might have developed tachyphylaxis, namely a diminished response to a drug requiring a larger dose for the same effect for example.

I know that my weight ballooned during the time I practiced as a GP prior to running, and that the weight fell off as I started exercising and eating less. This was no magic bullet, just common sense. The more I ran, keeping my eating constant, the more weight I lost. Keeping the running constant and drastically eating less and my weight dropped alarmingly.

I do realise that it isn't everyone who is as driven as I am and to push the boundaries isn't for everyone. Snacking on refined sugars clearly needed to be avoided and it wasn't difficult to differentiate between refined carbohydrates and good carbs.

My aversion to dairy products and animal fats and eventually meat, left me with fewer options. Hence my reliance on fish and vegetables such as avocados as a mainstay at meal times in the evening but really unsuitable for use throughout the day. This led me to the discovery of pure peanut butter as a staple during the day (and sometimes the night). I am happy to say that I have never tired of eating bottles of peanut butter through the years. I'd hate to hazard a guess how much I have consumed over the years. In 1977 while still in training, I ran16 km to work without having breakfast of course. On getting to work I discovered to my horror that there was no bread for lunch. I slipped out to the shops and bought a bottle of peanut butter and devoured it in one sitting. Even that never put me off my beloved peanut butter!

Prior to the onset of the argument regarding the cause of CHD, I had been eating a diet low in animal fats by personal preference. The fact that fat was thought to be detrimental was by the way. It wasn't the primary reason for me not eating fats. That they were thought to be bad was a bonus.

Dairy products were never a priority either and milk I though was for calves and not humans. As a result I never ate butter nor margarine or any other spreads. With large amounts of peanut butter, butter was superfluous. Neither did eggs appeal to me. However I have consumed them in one form or another. I always let my body dictate to my eating needs and as a rule, I only eat when hungry. I try to listen to my body but don't always succeed.

One occasion sticks in my mind I did listen to my body which said in no uncertain terms-"I NEED EGGS AND PLENTY OF THEM!" I had just finished paddling a 4 day, 240 km canoe race. I haven't yet written about my canoeing experiences and will describe this later in the epilogue(*2). The weather conditions were wretched and the last 60 km were paddled headlong into a gale in winter in the Cape Province of South Africa. At the finish I was thoroughly exhausted. Driving home I could not stop fantasising about eggs, I was craving them. On reaching home I boiled six eggs and gulped them down. If there were any more in the fridge I would certainly have eaten them too. I must have been so protein depleted to have induced such cravings.

An anecdote regarding my diet might surprise most. I must report my absolute aversion to garlic, something that is ubiquitous and found in most kitchens. My family and friends are fully aware of my idiosyncratic dislike or repulsion of garlic I'd go as far to say, but it isn't fully accepted by all and not everyone complies with my wishes regarding garlic. My wife uses it sparingly and takes pleasure in announcing that I wasn't aware of it after enjoying a splendid meal prepared by her. If I don't know its there I'm OK with that.

HOW WOULD I DESCRIBE MY EATING HABITS?

This has always been problem for me to describe as I don't really fit perfectly into any group. I'm not a true vegan because although I abstain from eating meat, I continue to eat fish and chicken. I also can't be regarded as a strict vegetarian, because they refrain from eating meat, dairy and eggs as well as all animal derived foods. Here too I break the rules because of my eating fish.

Could I be considered to eat the Paleo diet, similar to the diet eaten by pre historic man millions of years ago? Not really, because despite me eating vegetables, nuts and seeds and fruit, I don't eat meat as they certainly might have. As well as this the paleo's apparently exclude legumes and grains, something I eat a lot of. Therefore it is clear that slotting into one of these categories is pretty nigh impossible for me.

Looking around our kitchen at home, it becomes abundantly clear that virtually ever item in it is derived from plants, other than the refrigerated fish and chicken. There is one exception and that is a block of cheese, tucked away in a corner of the fridge and a carton of low fat milk, for use when visitors arrive for tea. That's it!

Simply stated, my eating habits can be classed as being a PLANT BASED DIET WITH FISH AND CHICKEN added in.

MY RATIONALE IN TRYING TO MAKE SENSE OF THE DIETRY QUAGMIRE

Traditional thought regarding the cause of CHD has never been challenged like it is today. The Keys cholesterol theory has been maligned by many quarters who want to replace it by bringing in sugars as the leading cause of heart disease.

I ask the question-why is it that certain families who

suffer from hyper cholesterolemias, have the propensity for dying relatively early from myocardial infarction? Surely some lipid fraction must be implicated?

We know that cholesterol is manufactured in the body and plays a vital role such as maintaining cell wall integrity, the manufacture of steroid hormones, and vitamin D. Why, one can ask, would a naturally occurring substance in the body be responsible for being potentially so destructive? Does ingested cholesterol have a different effect in the body or any effect at all? To the best of my knowledge these questions have not been answered.

Let us assume for a moment that, according to the new thinking, that cholesterol has nothing to do with CHD and that the blame lies fully with sugar. Sugar intake is meant to cause inflammation in the walls of the arteries which leads to damage and subsequently to plaque and thrombus formation. At post mortem examination it will be seen that plaques buildup, called atherosclerosis in most cases is present, of which cholesterol is a component. Known risk factors for atherosclerosis are hyperlipidaemia, hyperglycaemia, and smoking. Here we see that high fats and high blood sugar are thought to be contributory.

Why then are the antagonists so keen to scrap the hyperlipidaemia theory and only accept the high blood sugar theory, in which insulin resistance now apparently is the most important cause? Cholesterol is seen at post mortem to be part of the lesion, how can it not be implicated?

I take umbrage with this idea that it is acceptable to give diabetics carte blanche to eat saturated fats but only restrict carbohydrates. Giving saturated fats to patients with diabetes who develop micro vascular angiopathy is outrageous. Cutting out refined sugars in these patients is mandatory-nobody will argue with this.

There is an elephant in the room that nobody is seeing or refuse to discuss for what ever reason. This is not a zero-sum game, where one is right and therefore the other wrong. We need rather to take a middle path in dealing with the problem. I accept fully that refined sugar should be avoided and that insulin resistance is of cardinal importance in both diabetes and CHD, but I'm not prepared ignore the possibility of fats being implicated in the CHD. This is wishful thinking, and I personally will continue to avoid both fats and refined sugars where possible.

Here I stick my neck out again. Dietary advice is not something I willingly espouse because there is always someone out there who will refute one's ideas. People from a wide spectrum, ranging from dieticians to fringe loons who do very nicely from their vested interest in food fads, as well as supplements, lead to the inevitable outcome of disinformation. The problem is that many of these dietary ideas are unproven and then taken as gospel by the wider public. Observational, rather than interventional studies often form the basis of information which finds its way into reputable medical and scientific journals. There are many examples of this which I don't want to get into right now.

With regard to the LCHF diet and its application to diabetes my concerns are as follows: lowering carbohydrate intake is clearly a sensible option for type-1 diabetics and has been shown to make it easier to reduce the post meal glucose spikes with insulin, but wether this in itself independently reduces microvascular complications seen in diabetics is not known. What is known is that a very low carbohydrate diet may actually increase the risk of keto-acidosis.

Regarding type-2 diabetes, serious co-morbidities are cardio-vascular incidents such as stroke which often accompany the condition. Familial dyslipidaemias, obesity, insulin resistance and hypertension may be the important underlying factors in the development of stroke etc proving the importance of glucose control per se as well as well as control of abnormal lipids, being quintessential in preventing complications. The problems are complex and there is no 'quick fix' as yet!

The bottom line in this regard is that a LCHF diet may inadvertently effect the lipid profile the effects of which have not yet been studied in controlled clinical trials.

Should everyone be on a low CHO (controlled carbohydrate) diet? This question I asked a prominent diabetic specialist who answered as follows: I suppose it depends on what you wish to gain-better teeth perhaps, better marathon performance, fewer cases of Alzheimer's, quieter children, etc. Much of these purported benefits exist in the eye of the believer and are conjectural at worst and observational at best, (ie hypothesis generating but not proof). However, the noise made by the pundits that shriek that this is an inherently healthier diet than any other will really have to do some serious systematic studies to persuade me that an 'ideal' diet exists. Thus far this has not been the case. The best diet is the one you like!

This coming from one extremely well informed and versed in the management of diabetes over a life time, tells me more than I need possibly to know, and leaves me feeling happy with my own gut feeling regarding my diet. I feel more confident in actually recommending my diet, when asked about my thoughts on the so-called LCHF diet.

I have documented my physical and blood chemistry parameters for many years, and kept a strict watch over them. I have also remained cognisant of advances and new ideas. I am aware that what works for me might not be a panacea for all. I would never be so bold as to claim this. There is no one size fits all when searching for the perfect diet. I have chosen what works for me. I am always surprised when I read anything concerning causation of diabetes where carbohydrates and lipids are at loggerheads. Surely it is time to accept that both might be involved and that judicious avoidance of either plus a good dose of exercise might go a long way in helping to quell the epidemic.

EPILOGUE

SO WHAT CONCLUSIONS CAN I DRAW FROM MY RUNNING EPIPHANY?

Has my life changed since taking up running?

In one word-*undoubtably*. I underwent a metamorphosis mentally, physically, and spiritually. My entire outlook on life changed drastically. More important was the effect on my family, and in particular my son Graeme who turned out to be an elite canoeist, representing South Africa 14 years in a row. He won the first world cup in surf skiing in 2004.

I had become somewhat disenchanted with running races with the hype and TV coverage that became part of the running scene. To me running was a spiritual experience and the noise and business-like atmosphere that prevailed at races was not what I enjoyed any longer. I decided to look for a pastime that would bring me back to nature and at the same time be a challenge. Running would always be my favourite pastime but canoeing it was hoped would add another dimension to life.

I put my son Graeme in a canoe at age 9 years and he never looked back after that. The enjoyment never wore off and it turned out to be the perfect sport for him. This led to an interest in life saving which I encouraged as I used my anaesthetic skills to teach airway management to the young life savers of the Cape, making sure that they could save lives if called upon to do so.

Graeme at age 15 years, successfully captained the South African junior life saving team to Australia in 1987 and continued to travel to many countries partaking in world canoeing events.

At the time of writing this, Graeme's children taking after their father, with Hanna, the oldest at 10 years of age is winning medals in canoeing, is becoming an accomplished horsewoman, as is her younger sister Sky.

My dietary habits seemed to have been adopted by my son and his daughters. Milk and eggs are still part of their diet unlike mine, but time will tell. Interestingly enough they seem to have inherited some of my genes, we are all tall and it would seem that they are getting taller. I am 193 cm tall, and my son 196 cm. His 10 year old daughter was far ahead of the top percentile at age 2 years. It is said that one can double the hight of the child at age 2 to see what height the child should be as an adult. It could be interesting to see if this transpires.

WHAT PROOF DO I HAVE THAT MY IDEAS ON EXERCISE AND DIET HAVE BEEN SUCCESSFUL?

To date, I have been relatively healthy regarding chronic illnesses. I had all the children viral illnesses, with respiratory infections most common during my early years. At age 6 years I had bilateral viral pneumonia. In 1990 as an adult I had hepatitis-A, which stopped my Two Oceans 56 km career in its tracks. My liver enzymes were greatly increased and took 12 weeks to get back to normal. It was a sobering time.

Since that time I have kept a record of any blood work I have done over the years. Over this 30 year period, I am pleased to say that my lipid profile has remained well within normal limits, as have my kidney functions, and blood glucose levels. How much is genetic and how much from my lifestyle, I don't know. I wouldn't hazard a guess. What I will say is that this has worked for me and therefore see no reason to start changing my diet for diets like the Keto-diet, or low carbohydrate/high fat diet.

To the above I can add that my blood pressure has remained normal and therefore I have never had to treat it.

I mentioned earlier in the book that I used to have a resting pulse rate of around 35/min for years. This caused me to live with a range of arrhythmias which caused no problems till 2020, when I suddenly had several runs of ventricular tachycardia over a three month period, forcing me to have an ablation for the VT, followed by insertion of a pace maker, limiting my resting pulse rate to 50/min, which resolved the long standing bradycardia and multiple arrhythmia.

The big question was and is—what caused this VT? In my case, the electrophysiologists working on me were satisfied that the source which they successfully ablated was very localised. What caused it, they were not certain.

Having clearly become interested in cardiac electrophysiology, I have been reading vastly on the subject. It is starting to become clear that if exercise is good for one, then twice as much might not necessarily be twice as good. The opposite may be true and it looks that the evidence is mounting in this respect. Doing the sort of heavy milage we did over the years could be responsible for overstretching and therefore leading to scarring of the heart muscle. If this is the case then it's too late for me, the damage is done. I can only hope that the scarring if any remains limited.

I remain optimistically hopeful that my myocardium is healthy. I had an CT angiogram of my heart in 2015 (my age was 71 at the time, and this was repeated during the ablation I underwent in November 2020) which showed them to be patent, with a calcium score of 8, which is low for someone of 78 years of age.

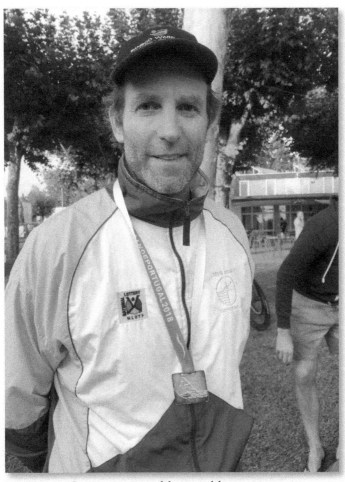

Graeme wins gold at world canoeing
marathon for veterans in Portugal 2018

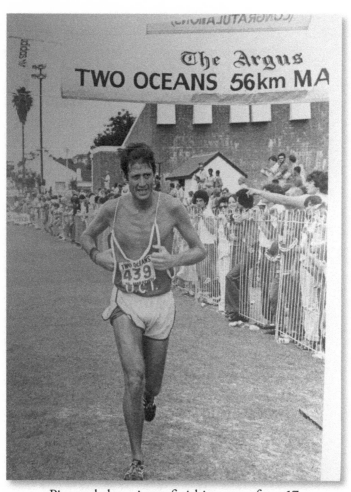

Pictured above is me finishing one of my 17
Two Oceans marathons in Cape Town with
not too much body fat in evidence

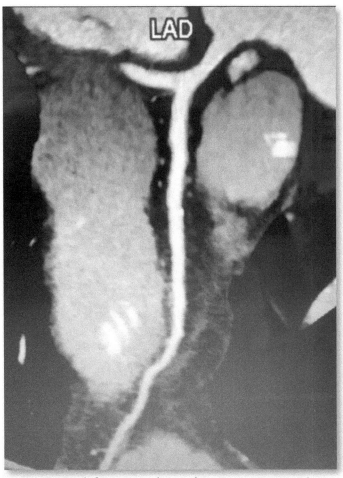

My LAD (left anterior descending coronary artery) -
Calcium score 8-low for a male over 70 years of age

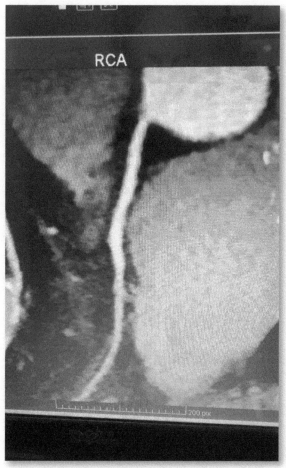

Angiogram of my heart showing the RCA (right coronary artery), taken in 2015 (calcium score of 8)

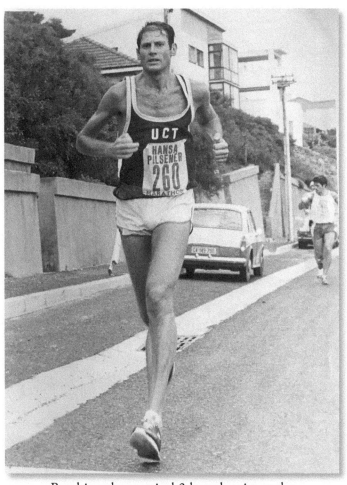

Breaking the mystical 3 hour barrier at the
Peninsula Marathon 1978 (2:52)

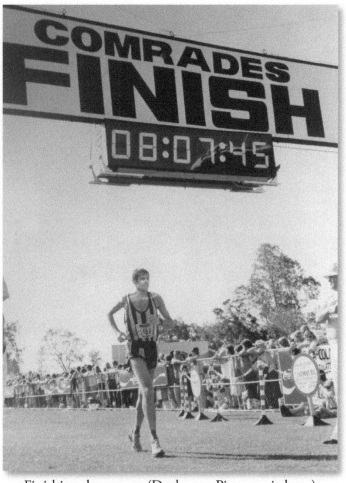

Finishing the up run (Durban to Pietermaritzburg)
Comrades marathon in a reasonable time

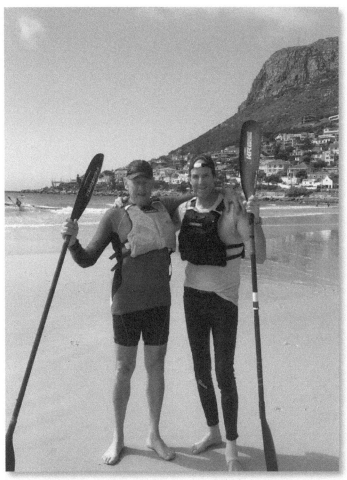

Graeme and I just having paddled the Light
House race in False Bay - a mere 16 kms jaunt

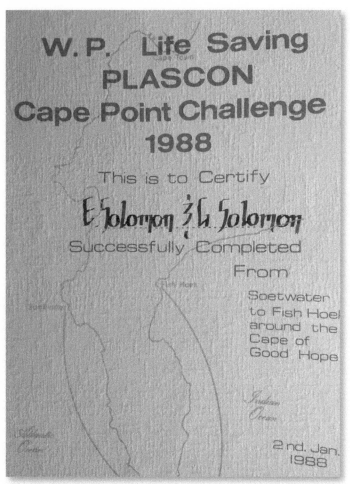

W. P. Life Saving
PLASCON
Cape Point Challenge
1988

This is to Certify

E Solomon & L Solomon

Successfully Completed

From

Soetwater
to Fish Hoel
around the
Cape of
Good Hope

2 nd. Jan.
1988

Certificate of having finishing the 1988 Cape Point
Challenge(65 Km) with my son aged 14 years

MY FINAL THOUGHTS

My final thoughts are that one needs a goal in life and needs to be focused on reaching this goal. Nothing supersedes good health in life and one must never loose sight of this. Everything else is of secondary importance. In todays world where we are facing unprecedented challenges, the loss of jobs, the devastation of the Covid pandemic, and generally the world seemingly out of control. What is of cardinal importance is remaining healthy in order to face up to these challenges.

Moses ben Maimon, (1138–1204), a well known medieval Jewish philosopher, instinctively knew then that exercising in the morning before eating was good for the body. Thinking about this the obvious conclusion can only be that the body utilises its own resources, namely mobilising glycogen stores from the muscles and liver before it has a chance to digest food recently taken in. Intermittent fasting is a continuation of this idea.

Did I ever tire of running per se? Most definitely not! Sure I used to get physically tired after strenuous exercise, but once the feeling of tiredness wore off, I was back into it again. It took me many years to start listening to my body but after many years of 'over doing' it, I finally obeyed. I learned to know my body well. I could divide tiredness into three categories, namely: tiredness of the legs, tiredness of the respiratory and cardiovascular system, and finally, tiredness of the head, feeling that I had not quite woken up yet which was often the case as I used to rise early in order to fit in a run before work.

In retrospect what would I do differently?

I would not have run as much as I did, limiting long runs to half marathons and less. The ultra marathons are not a good idea and many running friends have paid the price with knee and hip replacements. I was fortunate to have my knees and hips still in good shape, although my feet have taken a bit of a hammering, but nothing needing any special intervention.

As a result I infrequently go for a 3-4 km jog, but no more. I've taken up riding a mountain bike which affords me the opportunity to get good cardiovascular training without the pounding of my body. We live in the countryside where there are plenty of challenging hills to ride, all on gravel roads as I am wary of traffic. Fortunately the traffic is very light in the Swedish countryside in any event.

My wife and I have kayaks and paddle in summer on our lake which is 45 km long, so no shortage of things to do.

As Bertrand Russell, the British philosopher and intellectual (1872—1970) stated —"The more things you can do, the better". I love that statement and have applied it my whole life. The more, the merrier! So when I'm not running or walking or hiking or riding my bike or swimming, I read and play the fiddle.

WHERE DOES THIS ALL LEAVE US?

If the truth be told, the public at large must surly be confused regarding what is considered a healthy diet as well as the appropriate use of medications for the two medical problems of diabetes and cardiovascular disease. People no longer trust science or medicine, which is understandable as it is becoming evident that even the most prestigious of medical and scientific journals are prone to either faulty statistical analysis, or plagiarism or outright criminal behaviour publishing data which is tainted.(see *1) There are many examples of obfuscation at present, one such example being the use of Statins. It is difficult to know whether they are beneficial or not, or whether they do more harm than good. We hear than big Pharma is only interested in making a profit and nothing else. Every research article ends with conflict of interest, and it should be clear if funding was at all from big pharmaceutical companies. I as a medical doctor don't know what to believe any longer. I therefore decided to write this book in the hope of bringing a bit of common sense to the party.

It is not rocket science to see that type 2 diabetes and weight gain can be managed by a determined reduction in total carbohydrates, and specifically refined sugars. What is more contentious is the amount of total fats eaten. I propose a reduction in saturated animal fats to an absolute minimum, as well as avoiding triglycerides. Good fats in the form of fish omega 3 oils, and plant based oils from nuts and seeds and avocados are in abundance and are preferred.

Bashing carbohydrates and letting fats off the hook in coronary artery disease is not yet fully accepted world wide.

Insulin resistance and glucose intolerance surely is not the entire story. I find it hard to believe according to some sources, that doctors apparently have been hoodwinked for decades into believing that cholesterol and other fats cause heart disease. The narrative is gaining traction amongst the gullible This recent paradigm shift in thinking has created a polarisation amongst practitioners often leading to incendiary rhetoric. It has left confusion in its wake. I find it astounding that these so-called experts put the blame fully on carbohydrates as the cause for diabetes and heart disease. I am yet to hear from them regarding the possible harm caused by the cavalier intake of trans and saturated fats on the cardiovascular system as well as the peripheral micro-vasculature. Don't forget that the pathology of diabetes involves the small vessels. I await the scientific proof of the lack of casualty of cardiovascular pathology by fats, I am not holding my breath.

I fear it will be a while yet before we know the answer. Meanwhile I'm happy to watch the passing show and continue with my diet and exercise regime.

My dictum I live by is as follows:

I HAVE THE NEXT TEN MILLION YEARS TO LIE STILL-NOW IS THE TIME TO MOVE!

END

NOTES

(*1)

'TURTLES ALL THE WAY DOWN' vaccine science and Myth.(Edited by Zoey O'Toole and Mary Holland) References can be downloaded for this book from https://tinyurl.com/TurtlesBookEngRef

(*2)

I have only briefly mentioned my canoeing experiences. I did this not to detract from my running saga. I became interested in canoeing during the early 80's because I was looking for a change from distance running as I had more or less reached all my goals, as well as needing a break from the now extremely popular and much advertised and commercialisation running scene.

Running was still enjoyable but I no longer enjoyed the marathons which had become commercial events rather than simply running for the love of it. I therefore looked for an alternative, not to replace running, but to compliment it in away which allowed me to enjoy nature without the noise and hype of the big races.

Canoeing on rivers gave me exactly what I wanted, for a few years at least until canoeing too became a huge industry as well. Fortunately I partook in canoeing and surf ski events when they were in their infancies. I did many river races and marathons over several years, but my interest lay in watching my son Graeme go from a kid of 9 years when I first put him into a canoe, to representing South Africa as a Springbok canoeist for 14 years as well as a junior Springbok life saver, captaining the team over in Australia. He won the surf ski World Cup in April 2004. He continues to excel to this very day, having won gold as a veteran at the world canoeing marathon championships in Portugal in 2018.

(*3)
Y. Harari. Sapiens-a brief history. p78

ABOUT THE AUTHOR

Eric Solomon was born in South Africa during the Apartheid era. He was schooled in the Transvaal and qualified as a doctor in 1968 from the University of Pretoria (MB.Ch.B). He worked briefly in London after completing his internship and spent five years in general practice in Benoni, South Africa. He then moved to Cape Town where he completed his specialisation as an anaesthetist obtaining the FFA(SA) in 1977. He was on the staff of the famous Groote Schuur Hospital for 14 years, where Prof Barnard performed the first heart transplant. He then left to work in Israel for 8 years, after which he spent 10 years as an anaesthetic consultant in Ireland prior to moving to Sweden in 2010 working briefly till his retirement.

He retains a keen interest in medicine and anaesthetics but spends his time, riding his trail bike, canoeing on the nearby lake, hiking the pristine forests, reading and playing the fiddle with a group for fun and sometimes entertainment. He lives with his wife Eva-Lis and their golden retriever Dougal in the Swedish countryside.

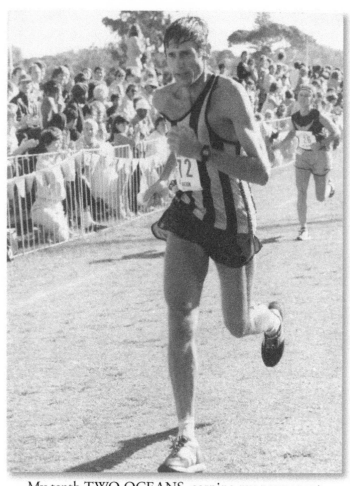

My tenth TWO OCEANS, earning my permanent
race number 25, a very proud and memorable
day. Most probably my best race ever! (1985)